From Fat to Fit

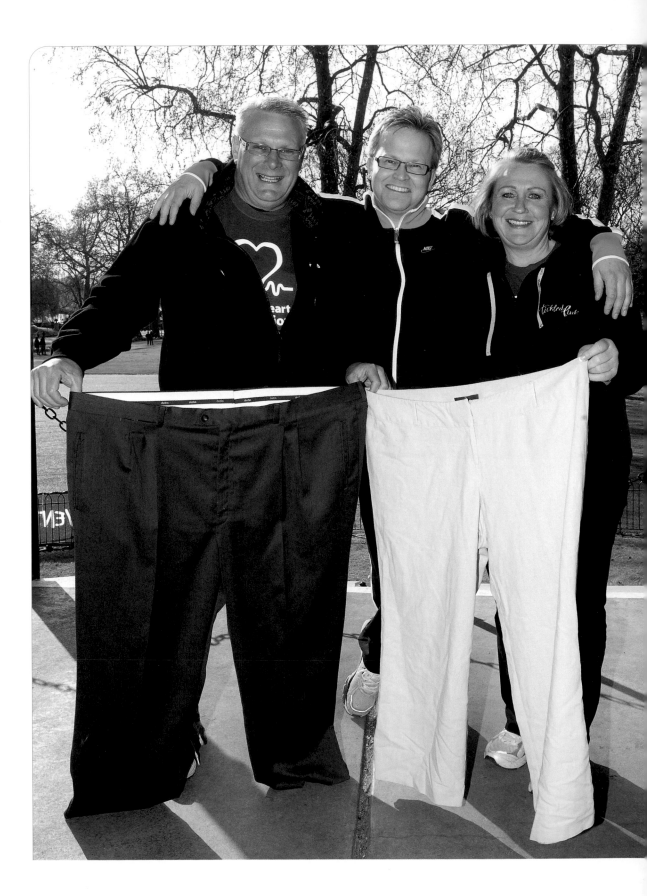

From Fat to Fit

The simple way to transform your family's health

**Outline Productions
with Sally Morris**

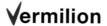

10 9 8 7 6 5 4 3 2 1

Published in 2011 by Vermilion, an imprint of Ebury Publishing

Ebury Publishing is a Random House Group company

The Random House Group Limited Reg. No. 954009

Addresses for companies within the Random House Group can be found at www.rbooks.co.uk

A CIP catalogue record for this book is available from the British Library

The Random House Group Limited supports The Forest Stewardship Council (FSC), the leading international forest certification organisation. All our titles that are printed on Greenpeace-approved FSC-certified paper carry the FSC logo. Our paper procurement policy can be found at www.rbooks.co.uk/environment

Colour reproduction by Dot Gradations Ltd, UK
Printed and bound by Firmengruppe APPL, aprinta druck, Wemding, Germany
Designed and typeset by Estuary English

ISBN 978 0 09 193947 2

Copies are available at special rates for bulk orders. Contact the sales development team on 020 7840 8487 for more information.

To buy books by your favourite authors and register for offers, visit www.rbooks.co.uk

The information in this book has been compiled by way of general guidance in relation to the specific subjects addressed, but is not a substitute and not to be relied on for medical, healthcare, pharmaceutical or other professional advice on specific circumstances and in specific locations. Please consult your GP before starting a diet or new fitness regime. So far as the author is aware the information given is correct and up to date as at August 2010. Practice, laws and regulations all change, and the reader should obtain up-to-date professional advice on any such issues. The authors and publishers disclaim, as far as the law allows, any liability arising directly or indirectly from the use, or misuse, of the information contained in this book.

Picture credits
All photography © Outline Productions, except on the following pages:
Front cover (left), back cover, 6, 32, © Sky1/Andi Southam; 14–16, 18, 19, 22, 25, 49, 50, 52–57, 62, 65, 66, 68, 73, 75, 80–84, 90, 94, 97–113, 117, 118, 122, 124–130, 150–152, 160–164, 170 (bottom), 179, 184–193, 206–208, 211, © istockphoto; 168 © defd – dfd Deutscher Fotodienst GmbH/Alamy; 175 © Image Source/Alamy; 181 © Justine Evans/Alamy; 209 © Cultura/Alamy; 170 (top) © Andres Rodriguez/ Alamy

Contents

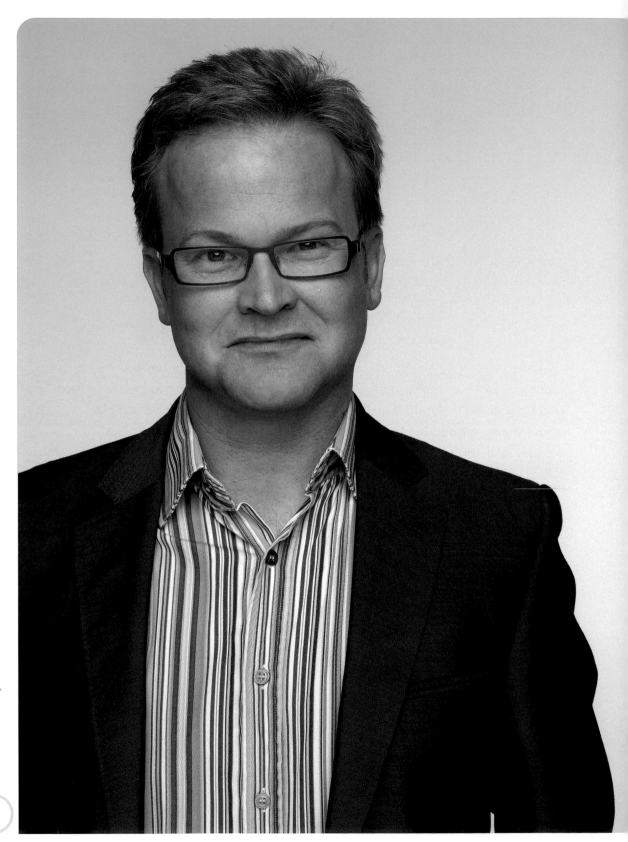

Foreword

AS A SUCCESSFUL, straight-talking motivator, it was ten years ago that I developed my no-nonsense weight-loss programme, having battled the bulge myself. I soon realised that a bit of practical common sense, combined with tough love, was the best way to melt that lard. I had tried all the fad diets, and local weight-loss groups only made me more depressed about being fat as I listened to the moans and groans of those who had failed to lose a pound that week. Yes, getting fatter wasn't nice, but tea and tissues would only delay things, and feeling sorry for myself would do nothing except turn me into an even bigger fatty.

Losing weight by eating less, eating better and moving more became my mantra and at the heart of it all was the big 'A' – Attitude! It had to be positive and I monitored it closely. If ever there was a day I felt I couldn't be bothered, I gave myself a good big kick up the bum and got back on the weight-loss wagon. With this approach I soon lost three stone, and as my confidence returned, I made the conscious decision I would never return to Fatsville.

Getting fat is so easy these days, with cheap junk food being sold on every corner, the vast majority of us owning a car, driving to the newsagent's five minutes' walk up the road and more and more of us shopping online rather than going for a good old walk! But can we really blame the availability of cheap chocolate, crisps, pizzas and fatty ready meals? After all, it is we who decide to eat it.

Sadly, as the years have gone by, we have as a society fallen into big fat habits and the real secret to a slimmer, trimmer figure is in breaking them. The good news is that these fatty habits can be melted as we form new healthy ones. In reality there can be no excuses, because what do excuses keep us? Fat!

With personal experience in the bag and a professional track record of helping those who had suffered years of living life in the fat lane, I was asked to present my own TV show, *Fat Families*, for Sky1HD and Sky1. Working with families as opposed to individuals was to be a real challenge but one that I would relish; bring it on, I thought!

Experience, of course, told me it was a task in itself to change the life of an individual, so how on earth was I going to tackle the complexities of a family? But with sleeves rolled up and with that all-important positive attitude, I was determined to help my families get the result they wanted as the war on fat commenced. And I did just that, seeing family members shed anything from one stone to over four stone in just twelve weeks.

Now, working with fat families all over the UK, I have grown to love the weekly challenge that the families and I face. From the start I encourage the family to work as a team; there's nothing better than working as a family unit as opposed to trying to ditch the fat all by yourself. Being completely honest with each other is another of my ground rules. Brushing things under the carpet and turning your back on the truths spell danger.

I recall fondly James Joell-Ireland, who eventually owned up to having curry on toast! It's no wonder that week he didn't lose so much weight. With ground rules in place I crack on with the families, turning around a fat-friendly lifestyle to one that steers them in the opposite direction to Tubby Town.

Immediately getting the families to face up to the truth about their fatty lifestyle, I arrange for them to get medically checked out as well as getting up close and personal with the reality of how fat they actually are. (You should always consult your GP before embarking on a weight-loss plan.)

The truth does hurt but it's critical to have a reality check before my fat-busting interventions begin. This part of the journey was particularly painful for the Huzzeys and Haddrells but it immediately motivated them to take action and start losing weight. I encourage you all to confront your lifestyle before developing a plan of action to ditch the fat. Do you spend too long on the sofa? Do you spend too much time nibbling on high-sugar snacks? Does your attitude need an MOT? If the answer is YES to any of these, then make a decision right now to do something about it.

On the show we helped the families lose weight by shock tactics and a number of interventions designed to meet the needs of each individual.

This included a tailored nutrition plan, exercise regime and a number of motivational tools – all of which are detailed in this book.

Creativity is always critical when I help the families to lose weight – one size does not fit all. Take the Huzzeys, who weren't particularly inspired by the gym but adored Bollywood dancing, and the Haddrells, who went bonkers for aquaaerobics. Taking the first step into exercise is difficult for many, but once that step is taken you will never look back. Both Neil and Toni Blackholly are testament to that. After years of sitting on a sofa eating, and eating more, it is now not unusual for them to run five miles and look forward to the next! The same goes for food, and with the help of the recipes and meal plans outlined in this book you will mix and match what works for you and your family.

I do hope you find this book a tool that kick-starts your family's weight loss and that you all begin to say goodbye to fat and hello to fit.

Remember, what's most important is to maintain that positive attitude and enjoy the journey. So NO EXCUSES! You deserve it.

– Steve Miller

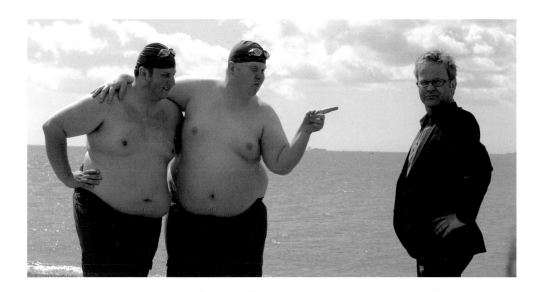

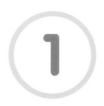

Taking the first steps to becoming fitter families

If you've opened this book, we hope it's because you're ready to take the first step in changing your family's eating and lifestyle habits; to lose weight, get fitter and feel better — as a family.

And the aim of this book is to help you see that this change isn't all about going without, about giving up treats and enduring punishing, dull exercise regimes — it's about looking at life a bit differently, asking yourself a few questions and breaking out of old habits.

If you follow the suggestions in this book you should not only lose weight and feel healthier, but you're also likely to feel happier, more confident and see the results of your efforts in more active, more outgoing children.

If you've watched motivational coach (and former fatty) Steve Miller build a relationship with the families he's worked with on the TV show *Fat Families*, you'll know that finding your own reasons to lose weight is the key to success — it's much harder to keep strong when you're doing something just because you've been told to by other people.

But when you read this book we think you'll find lots of reasons to make changes — obviously your family's health being the most important one.

In modern life it can be hard to stay in shape. We're all busier than we used to be and there's nothing more tempting than a ready-made meal or a takeaway when you come home from work or when you're feeling an energy slump. Shopping centres encourage us to use lifts or escalators, not stairs; busy roads put many people off cycling or letting younger children play outside; and everywhere you look, at any time of day, there's food on offer. Food, sadly, that's often packed with fat and sugar or hidden dangers such as lashings of mayonnaise on a salad sandwich. Food that pretends to be slimming by using the label 'low fat'.

Look along your supermarket shelves and see how many foods have a 'low-fat' version. What they won't tell you is that fat carries much of the flavour in foods and makes it feel good in our mouths, so if you take it out you often need to replace it with something else. And that something else is often sugar.

Low-fat breakfast cereals are often packed with sugar, so even as we try to cut back on one 'bad' foodstuff, we are tricked into taking in another.

And we're eating far more than we need to. When we were labouring in fields all day or doing all the housework without any electrical appliances, we needed lots of high-energy foods to keep us going. The high calories in a traditional English breakfast were important for a man doing hard physical labour, rather than a luxury.

But now most of our lives are inactive; for many of us in sit-down jobs, the only exercise we get is walking to and from the car. And if we're at home all day, many of us drive the kids to school, drive to the supermarket and often don't walk further than up a flight of stairs.

So we don't usually need high-energy foods, or even as much food on our plates as we like to think. Instead, we're eating because we like it – we like the taste of sweet and fatty foods so we stop listening to our bodies and stop waiting until we sense hunger pangs to trigger us into eating what we need.

So, if you recognise that you're one of those people who has allowed the weight to creep on, who prefers watching sport to playing it, and snacking all day to eating well-balanced meals – remember that you're passing these habits on to your children and it's already affecting their long-term health.

The sciencey bit

How can you tell the difference between when you're genuinely hungry and when you're just eating because you fancy a chocolate bar?

Genuine hunger tends to build slowly; it's a physical sensation of emptiness that goes away when you eat something – whether that's an apple or a doughnut. And if you're really hungry, you'll happily grab an apple!

Emotional hunger, or craving, comes on more suddenly and it's usually a desire for a particular food – so if someone offered you an apple, you'd turn it down because you really want chocolate. This sort of hunger usually hits when you're feeling bored, grumpy or miserable, and is simply a desire for something sweet and fatty because it will give your brain instant pleasure.

Although we think our stomach dictates our appetite, it's actually controlled by hormones and peptides, which communicate between the brain and stomach.

The main hunger hormone is called ghrelin, and it hits multiple parts of the brain to stimulate us to eat.

When we've eaten and are pleasantly full, the nerves that detect our stomach stretching send a message to the brain to say we've had enough and the stomach decreases the movement of food down into the intestines until there's more room down there. This explains why our stomach can still feel full a long time after having a big meal. Then another hormone, leptin, suppresses the appetite trigger until we are genuinely hungry again.

The problem with this finely balanced system is that it's actually very easy to override. We can choose to stop listening to our 'full' sensation because we get so much pleasure out of eating that we want to carry on doing it.

In fact, research in rats has shown that the pleasure centres in the brain develop the same sort of changes in response to sweet, fatty foods as cocaine addicts feel when they take the drug!

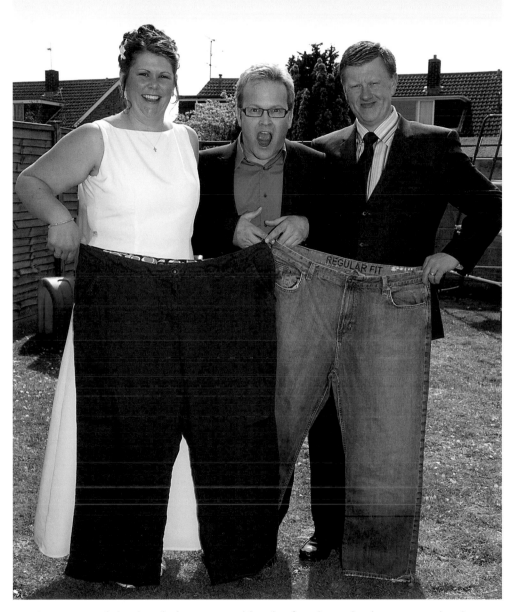

As you read this book, be inspired by the families who have completely changed their lives for the better by facing up to their bad habits and getting their entire families together in losing weight and getting fit.

Listen to the experts who will show you how you can turn your own lives around with a combination of willpower, support and a better understanding of what makes you fat and what makes you fit.

After all, you owe it to yourselves and to your children to enjoy a long and happy life.

2

How much should you weigh?

As more and more people become overweight it's easy to compare yourself to other people and think, 'I'm not as fat as most people in this room/street/office.' The problem is that as we grow fatter as a population, being overweight becomes more 'normal', so we don't actually notice how we're putting on weight because we don't stand out from the crowd.

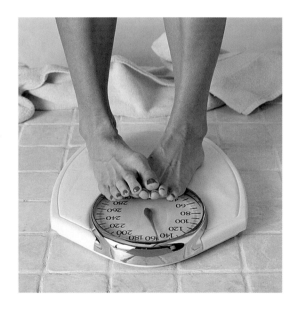

But there are several ways in which we can measure whether or not our weight is in a healthy, ideal range.

1. Adult Body Mass Index

The first of these is the Body Mass Index (BMI). It is a diagnostic tool that has been used for some time as a guide to what your weight range should be for your height. It's not perfect – people who are very muscular can sometimes seem to creep into an overweight bracket because muscle is denser than fat, so a rugby prop forward may be heavy for his height but isn't actually carrying excess fat, he's carrying dense muscle.

And as you age, you naturally lose muscle, so this can skew your results slightly. Also, some ethnic groups, for example people from South Asia, often have a lower amount of muscle and a higher fat ratio for the same BMI. But it's a useful calculation to start with.

Calculating your BMI

As accurately as you can, measure your height and weight and then do the following calculation. ⋯⋰

$$\frac{\text{Weight in kilograms}}{\text{Height in metres} \times \text{height in metres}} = \text{BMI}$$

You can use either metric (kilograms and metres) or imperial (pounds and inches) as long as both measurements use the same system. It may sound complicated but there are websites that can do the sum for you; try www.nhs.uk/tools or www.eatwell.gov.uk/healthydiet/healthyweight/bmicalculator.

For example, if you weigh 75 kg and stand 1.8 metres tall, then you'll perform the following calculation:

As you can see from the table below, that's nicely in the middle of the healthy weight range.

$$\frac{75}{1.8 \times 1.8} = 23.15$$

BMI range chart

BMI	Weight scale
Less than 18.5	Underweight
18.5–24.9	Healthy
25–29.9	Overweight
Over 30	Clinically obese

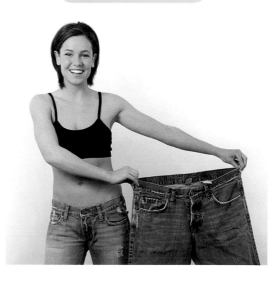

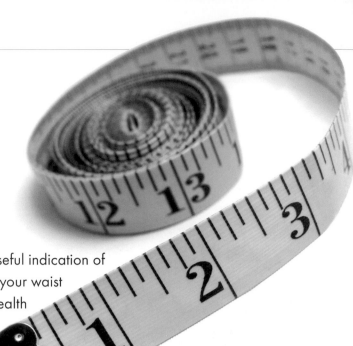

2. Waist size

A simpler and probably more useful indication of being overweight is to measure your waist size. This is because the latest health research has found that fat around the middle of your body is an indication of the level of fat being carried around the important organs inside your body, such as the liver and heart. So it's a measure not just of your external fat but also a sign of what's happening inside your body.

Women with a waist size of 88 cm (35 in) or more and men with a waist size of 102 cm (40 in) or more are most at risk of cardiovascular disease. There is an increased risk of the disease for women with measurements of more than 80 cm (32 in) and men whose measurement is over 94 cm (37 in).

If your waist measurement matches the above levels, you are putting yourself at risk of health conditions, such as type 2 diabetes and heart disease.

Apple or pear?

You can go one step further and calculate your waist to hip ratio to see how your waist size compares to the rest of your build.

Divide your waist measurement by your hip measurement.

$$\frac{\text{Waist measurement}}{\text{Hip measurement}} = \text{Waist to hip ratio}$$

It doesn't matter if you measure in centimetres or inches, but make sure that you use the same measurement for both your waist and hip. So a waist

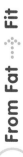

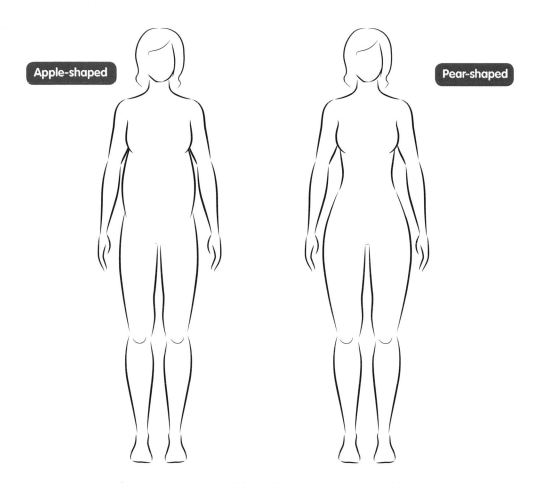

Apple-shaped

Pear-shaped

measurement of 33 inches divided by a hip measurement of 38 inches = 0.87. Again, there are online calculators available if you need help!

Ideally, the ratio should be no more than 0.85 for women and 1.0 for men. If your ratio is between 0.82 and 0.89, you are probably what's called 'apple-shaped'; if it's between 0.72 and 0.78, you are probably 'pear-shaped'.

In health terms 'apples' are more at risk of diabetes and cardiovascular disease than pears, but the good news is that because the weight is put on by eating the wrong food and exercising too little, it can be lost more easily by changing your diet and exercise habits.

'Pears', generally women, tend to put on weight around their hips and thighs, which can be more difficult to shift. But research shows it is less damaging for your health to have larger hips and more important to lose fat around the middle.

3. Body fat percentage

It's now possible to measure your body fat as a percentage of your total body weight – and monitor that as you lose weight; it's fat that's disappearing.

You can buy special scales that use electric currents to measure resistance in the muscles and fat, or you may find that your gym or GP's surgery has them. In the TV series *Fat Families*, Professor David McCarthy uses a special machine that can accurately measure just how much of your body is fat.

How much should my children weigh?

It's more difficult to have hard-and-fast rules about how much children should weigh. Boys and girls have different growth patterns and their size varies with growing periods so there's more variety.

Your doctor will have guidelines if you are worried that they're putting on weight.

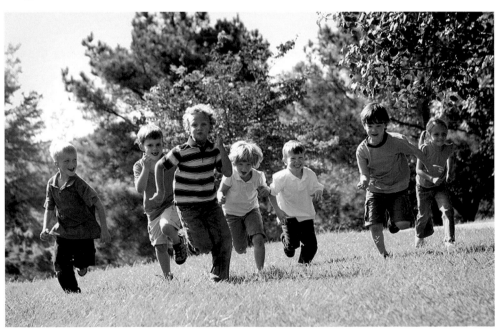

The most obvious thing is to look at them and see if they seem to be carrying any excess fat. Children should be active and physically fit and not get out of breath easily when playing or riding a bike.

They shouldn't have rolls of fat around their tummies or thighs. Try not to compare them to other people's children – it doesn't matter who they look like, you know your child best and can see if they seem to be outgrowing their clothes faster than they used to.

It's the same with children and adults – as a population there are now more overweight and obese children, so carrying excess weight appears normal and your child won't stand out.

The important thing is not to make a fuss about their weight. You can help them to change their eating habits by changing the way the whole family eats and behaves. If you start to nag them, they may start to eat in secret or develop eating problems.

You can, however, encourage your children to be more active through play, walking, riding their bikes or taking up a sport, and also limit the amount of time they spend in front of the TV or computer.

Lead by example!

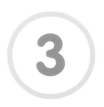

Why being fat is bad for your health

Professor David McCarthy of London Metropolitan University is an expert on nutrition, and body fat in particular. As a consultant on *Fat Families*, he worked with the families trying to lose weight and saw how changes in their lifestyle could bring about fairly dramatic weight loss. Even more important, families who change the way they live will keep the weight off, not end up in a cycle of 'yo-yo' dieting – losing weight/gaining weight – which is very bad for the body.

And because he works closely with families and children, Professor McCarthy knows that children with fat parents tend to get fat too – and this pattern is building up huge problems for the future. This is one of the main reasons why parents should listen to his advice and change the whole family's eating and exercise habits. As he says:

'Obesity is probably the biggest public health crisis in the UK. The older generation, raised during or just after the war, grew up on smaller meals, with limited access to sweet and fatty foods, but the generation growing up now are being raised on a totally different diet, and a totally different way of eating. The danger is that they will die at a younger age than their parents and certainly not live to the sorts of old age we are used to seeing in today's 80- and 90-year-olds.

'Obesity is creeping into childhood – we are seeing it start younger and younger, even in toddlers at the age of two – the growth in obesity among children is the largest of any age range.

'Forty years ago there may have been just one overweight child in an entire primary school class, and they were probably teased or bullied because they stood out from the crowd. The other kids were active and running around, and at weekends Mum probably had to call them in from playing outside to sit down for meals. But now, around 1 in 3 children of primary school age are overweight, or even obese, so they don't stand out quite so much. Our points of reference have changed, so parents will look at other kids in the playground who are just as overweight as theirs and not think they should do anything about it. And the chances are that Mum or Dad are also overweight but compare themselves to other overweight adults so don't feel they need to change.'

The two problems are lifestyle and personal responsibility. As a society, we simply eat too much – the portion sizes are too large, and we eat too often and too much of the wrong sorts of food.

FACT
The average waistband of two-year-old girls has increased by more than 5% in a decade, while that of boys has grown by 4%.

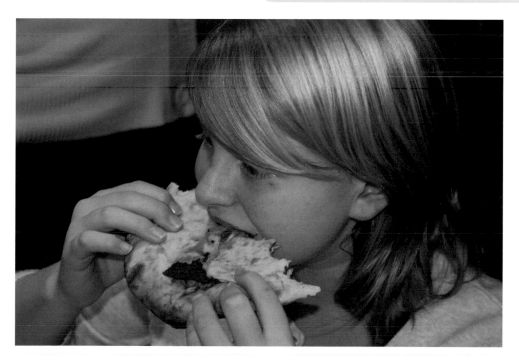

The food industry is also to blame. Food is cheap and plentiful – which should be a good thing – but what is widely available is mass-produced, calorie-dense food that's not only cheap but seriously unhealthy. It's possible to pick up a meal of fried chicken, chips and a fizzy drink for less than £5 – but it's packed full of fat and sugar.

Fizzy drinks are one of the worst culprits for obesity in children. We've seen how in America for some kids fizzy drinks are their main fluid intake. It used to be a rare treat for parties or meals out but now it's an all-day drink and there's nothing good in a cola drink – no nutrients at all.

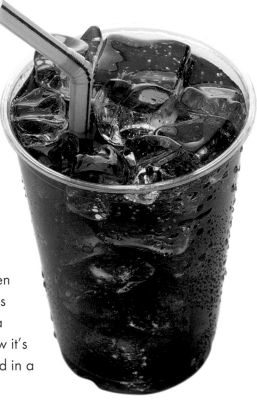

What our bodies need

Our bodies need us to eat regularly and to stop eating when we feel pleasantly full. To stay feeling full, the best choices are protein and complex carbohydrate – strangely, fat doesn't trigger our 'full' response in the same way, so starting the day with a whole-grain cereal will keep you going longer than a refined cereal. Some protein at breakfast – like eggs, for example – will also help stave off the mid-morning munchies.

Our bodies evolved as hunter-gatherers surviving on wild plants, berries, fruit and nuts with the occasional treat of a hunted animal – but that animal would have been wild and its meat would have been lean.

Our bodies learned to store fat because we didn't know when the next meal was coming – now we know the next meal will be along whenever we want it, so there's no need to store fat for the 'hungry' days. But our body's biology doesn't know that, so it stores anything we eat that we don't burn off in energy.

Our brains are also programmed to tell us to eat from as many different food sources as possible, to make sure we have the widest range of vitamins, minerals, proteins, fats and carbohydrates.

This is apparent when we have a three-course meal. We'll have a starter, maybe a soup, then we'll manage a main course, but if they brought out a second main course we wouldn't want it. But when they bring the dessert menu, we'll find room for a sweet pudding even though it's usually packed with calories, fat and sugar.

The health risks

Obesity affects every system in the body. It isn't just about what we look like on the outside, it's about the damage it's causing on the inside and there's no doubt at all that obesity kills.

Heart disease

Obesity is one of the major causes of heart disease. Heart disease is the biggest killer in the UK and, sadly, the main cause of death in people under 75. That level of premature death could be cut if obesity levels dropped.

Together, diseases of the heart and blood circulatory system, called cardiovascular disease, or CVD, cause more than 1 in 3 of all deaths in the UK – that's around 200,000 deaths a year. Heart disease may give you a heart attack or cause a stroke, and even if you don't die, you may be left disabled or with a very restricted life.

One of the main problems of cardiovascular diseases is that the arteries become blocked by a build-up of plaque, a sticky substance made up of cholesterol, calcium and blood platelets. Plaque sticks to the walls of the major blood vessels and slows down the flow of blood, sometimes stopping it altogether. When the heart muscle is deprived of oxygen – carried to it by the blood – it dies. Obesity can also cause the wall of the heart's left ventricle (the part that pumps blood around the body) to thicken so that it doesn't pump properly.

> **FACT**
> - **1 in 5 men and 1 in 7 women die from heart disease. This is about 250 people a day, or one person every six minutes.**
> - **Around 2.6 million people in the UK are living with heart disease.**
> - **Strokes cause around 53,000 deaths a year.**
> **(Figures from the British Heart Foundation.)**

High blood pressure

Your blood pressure is simply a measure of how hard your blood is pushing against the walls of your arteries (the blood vessels that carry blood away from the heart to all the tissues and cells in your body).

You'll notice that your doctor gives you two figures when taking your blood pressure, for example '120 over 80' (120/80): the first figure (systolic) is the pressure at which your heart beats and pushes the blood around your body; the second figure (diastolic) is when your heart rests in between beats.

Although readings can change depending on the time of day and external factors (for some, the stress of having their blood pressure taken actually makes their blood pressure rise!), your blood pressure is mostly constant.

Ideally it should be below 140/85 (around 120/70 in a young adult), but if you've already suffered from a stroke, heart attack or have heart disease, your doctor will want it to be lower than 130/80.

High blood pressure can run in families and is often treated by drugs, but in many cases it can be controlled by changing your diet and lifestyle. Losing

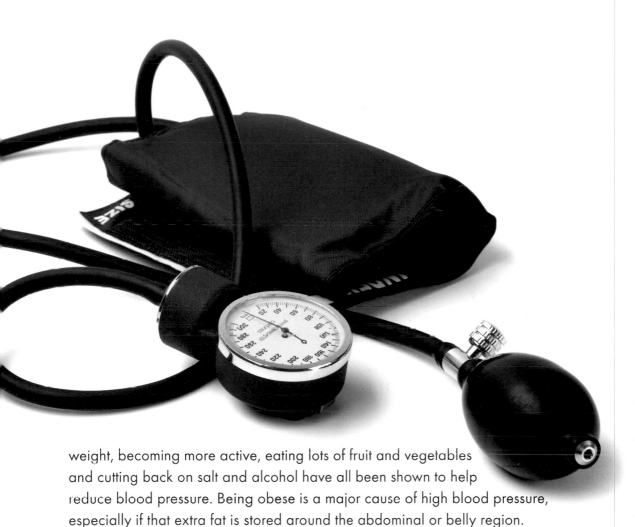

weight, becoming more active, eating lots of fruit and vegetables and cutting back on salt and alcohol have all been shown to help reduce blood pressure. Being obese is a major cause of high blood pressure, especially if that extra fat is stored around the abdominal or belly region.

In this country, a third of all adults – that's 16 million people (32% men to 29% women) – have high blood pressure and many of them don't even know they have it because often it shows no symptoms. That's why it's worth having your blood pressure checked when you visit your GP – it only takes a minute.

High blood pressure not only contributes towards heart disease and strokes, it damages your heart and blood vessels, and can also cause kidney disease, eye problems and certain types of dementia. It can be especially dangerous in pregnant women and can cause impotence in men by damaging the arteries that bring blood to the penis. So lots of reasons to get that blood pressure down!

Type 2 diabetes

There are two sorts of diabetes: type 1 and type 2. Type 1 develops when the body's insulin-producing cells (in the pancreas) have been destroyed and your body can't produce insulin. Insulin controls the cells' ability to take up glucose (a sugar) from the blood – if there's no insulin, the cells can't take up the glucose and it stays in your bloodstream.

Although type 1 diabetes can develop at any age it usually begins in younger life, often in early childhood. It can be treated by daily insulin injections and by maintaining a healthy, regular diet and regular exercise to keep the blood sugar stable. Only about 5 to 15% of people with diabetes have type 1.

> **FACT**
> The health risks increase as your blood pressure rises. Between the ages of 40 and 70, for every rise of 20 in your systolic reading or 10 in your diastolic reading, the risk of heart disease and stroke doubles (in the range of 115/75 to 185/115).

Type 2 diabetes (formerly known as maturity-onset diabetes) is a health time bomb in the UK. Over the next five to ten years, this disease will escalate and show itself in younger and younger people. It is caused by the body not making enough insulin and developing 'insulin resistance'. That means the insulin doesn't work properly and the body makes more and more insulin to compensate.

Although some South Asian and black ethnicities in this country are more prone to develop type 2 diabetes, it is appearing among the general population at a younger and younger age, whereas many years ago it used to be a disease seen mainly in older people.

We know that being overweight is the single biggest cause of type 2 diabetes and that people who carry most of their excess weight around their middle are most likely to develop the condition.

Once you have type 2 diabetes it is possible to control it through strict diet and exercise, but some people will have to take medicine. It is an avoidable disease for many people and losing weight is the most important step in heading it off.

Diabetes carries all sorts of additional health risks, including:

Cardiovascular disease

When the level of glucose in the blood isn't controlled for a long period it can affect the lining of the arteries, which, in turn, increases the risk of them becoming blocked, or 'furred'. Blocked arteries can lead to heart attacks and strokes.

People with diabetes often have low levels of the good sort of cholesterol, HDL (see page 31), which also adds to the risk of arteries becoming blocked.

Retinopathy

The eye is richly supplied with blood vessels but they are very narrow. People with diabetes are at risk of developing abnormal or leaky eye vessels, which can damage the retina. This can lead to sight problems and even blindness.

If you are diagnosed with diabetes, it is very important to have your eyes examined by an optician every year with a special camera. Diabetes is the biggest cause of blindness among adults.

Nerve damage (neuropathy)

Diabetes can damage the nerves that carry messages from the brain to the body, making your feet or hands numb or tingly, causing misshapen feet, weak muscles and your bladder to work less effectively. It can also cause impotence in men, as the penis finds it hard to maintain an erection. Diabetes is one of the leading causes of amputation of the lower limbs throughout the world.

Kidney disease (nephropathy)

Long-term diabetes can contribute towards kidney disease, although this isn't a common side complication. Diabetes damages the small blood vessels in and around the kidneys, so keeping blood-glucose levels as near to normal as possible is the best way to prevent kidney problems. It's also very important to keep blood pressure at normal levels when dealing with kidney complications.

Cancer

There is growing evidence that being overweight increases your risk of developing certain cancers, in particular breast, ovarian, uterine, prostate and colon (bowel) cancers. The link between obesity and bowel cancer appears stronger in men. In bowel cancer, the benefits of exercise are marked – regular physical activity reduces the risk of bowel cancer by up to 50%.

Liver damage

'Fatty liver' used to be seen in alcoholics only, but now we are seeing it in younger and younger patients, and it isn't related to what they drink. About 1 in 5 adults in the UK is thought to suffer from it, while 4 out of 5 obese adults do.

It is what it says: a build-up of fat within the liver cells, and in most cases it is linked to being overweight. The condition increases your risk of heart attacks and stroke, and in some people this build-up of fat can lead to serious liver problems, causing liver inflammation or the build-up of scar tissue (fibrosis). In the worst cases, a severe build-up of scar tissue replaces healthy liver cells and the liver stops being able to function properly, leading to cirrhosis and eventually liver failure.

Of course, heavy drinkers put themselves at even greater risk of liver disease.

Joint problems

Being overweight places unnatural strain on joints, which weren't built to take the extra load. Knees in particular can suffer, especially if you are bending down a lot, and overweight people have more than their share of cartilage tears.

Pregnancy problems

Being very overweight can affect women's chances of getting pregnant and in men, the production of enough healthy sperm.

The ovaries and, to a lesser extent, other glands such as the adrenal glands near your kidneys, produce the female reproductive hormone, oestrogen. But your body fat also produces some oestrogen, so the more fat you have, the more oestrogen is produced, disrupting the balance of your hormones and your monthly cycle.

Pregnant women who are heavily overweight are at increased risk of developing pregnancy diabetes, which can harm both the developing foetus and the mother. Babies of women with pregnancy or 'gestational' diabetes are often larger than other babies and run a higher risk of being born with jaundice or being delivered by Caesarean section. And overweight mothers risk suffering more complications if they deliver by Caesarean section.

FACT
Babies of obese mothers are 3.5 times more likely to be admitted to a neonatal intensive care unit than babies of healthy-weight mothers.

Recent studies have shown that overweight women are less likely to respond to IVF treatment and many NHS clinics refuse to offer fertility treatment to heavily overweight women for this reason.

Obesity also affects men's fertility levels. One recent study, carried out in 2008, showed that obese men were three times more likely to have a lower sperm count as men of the same age who were in the normal weight range. And their sperm quality was lower too. Those fat cells in men are producing the female hormone oestrogen (one of the reasons obese men develop 'man boobs'!), which may alter their hormone balance. And, as mentioned earlier, being overweight can damage a man's ability to maintain an erection.

Depression

Being very overweight doesn't just cause physical problems, it is also a major cause of depression and other mental health problems. Although we all know that people tend to comfort-eat when they are fed up, it's actually more scientific than that – as we see with infertility problems, obesity can alter the body's delicate hormone balance. And it works both ways – depressed people are more likely to become overweight, and overweight people are more likely to become depressed.

But taking steps towards tackling obesity can have two very positive effects on depression: not only are you working towards losing weight by cutting down on your food intake, which will make you feel better physically, you are also hopefully increasing your levels of physical activity, and this is now accepted as a very effective way of treating certain types of depression, because exercise raises the level of 'feel-good' chemicals in the body known as endorphins.

Cholesterol

If there's one thing most of us have learned from all the health information that we're bombarded with, it's that cholesterol, a sort of waxy fat carried in the bloodstream, is bad and that levels should be as low as possible. Well, that's about half right.

The truth is that we need cholesterol to make cell membranes and to help the body to perform many of its functions. But that cholesterol is carried around in the blood by lipoproteins, which come in two versions: High Density Lipoproteins (HDL) and Low Density Lipoproteins (LDL).

The HDL is considered to be good – it carries the excess cholesterol away to be processed out of the body by the liver. The LDL is bad, as it carries the cholesterol around the body to be used by cells but leaves any that is not used in the blood to clog up the arteries. So the best thing to have is a high level of HDL and a low level of LDL – and that's what your doctor will look for when he or she tests your blood for cholesterol.

Lowering cholesterol can be done, in part, by changing your diet. The most important change is to cut down on saturated fat (which the body uses to make cholesterol in the liver).

It is also beneficial to eat foods like good old-fashioned porridge, which contains a special sort of fibre that has been shown to lower the levels of bad cholesterol. There are other cholesterol-lowering foods on the market these days, such as some of the margarines and yoghurts that contain special plant extracts called stanols and sterols. Additionally, healthy fats, including omega-3 fats found in oily fish such as sardines, mackerel and tuna, can help to lower LDL, and olive oil is rich in a type of fat called monounsaturates. All these fats help keep your blood lipid levels within the healthy range.

In a normal person, the overall cholesterol level should be less than 5.0 mmol/l (millimoles per litre), with an LDL of 3.0 mmol/l, or lower. If you already have or are in a high-risk group for heart disease (for instance, if you are overweight or a smoker) you should aim for a lower level, less than 4.0 mmol/l overall, with an LDL of 2.0 mmol/l or less. Some people find that high cholesterol levels run in their family, so high cholesterol may not be down to their diet.

Changing your diet has a useful effect but may not do the whole job. Many people are advised to take drugs called statins that lower the levels of cholesterol.

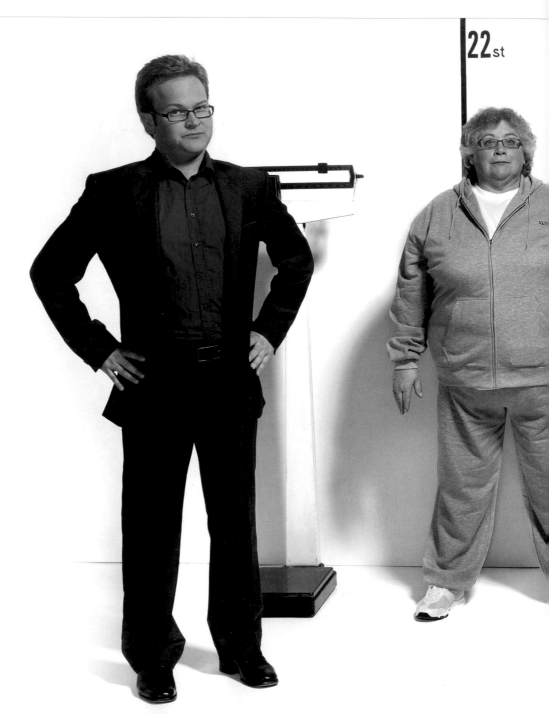

22st

Get started now!

So, that's all the bad news about why we want you to lose weight, get active and live longer! The good news is that once you start losing weight, many of these health conditions improve or stabilise fairly quickly. So it's never too late to chuck out the junk food and go for a walk in the park.

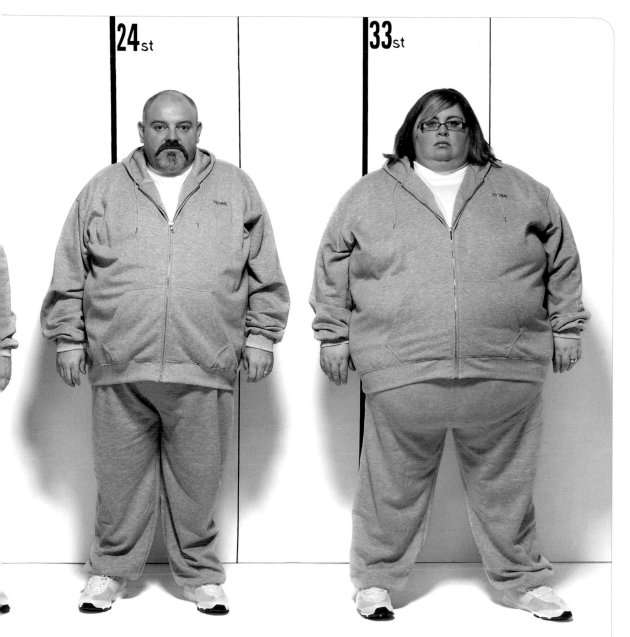

24st   33st

As you'll see from some of the inspirational families who are featured in this book, changing their lifestyle has allowed them to throw away some of their blood pressure, cholesterol and diabetes medications (with their doctor's approval, of course) as well as eased the pain in their joints. And their self-esteem and confidence have also improved, which are every bit as important as seeing changes in physical health.

It's given them a new lease of life and has also hugely improved their children's chances of growing up to live a longer, healthier life.

The Blackholly family from Wiltshire

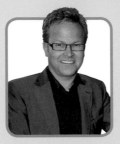

Steve visited the Blackhollys from Wiltshire.

'I met a right pair of podgy parents – the wobblers from Wiltshire – who'd been chomping away on junk food for the last ten years.

'This pair were cramming in a stomach-stretching 8,000 calories a day between them.

'And it's not just their own bellies they were stuffing with rubbish. The Blackholly bambinos were fast becoming Junior Junk Food Junkies.'

Neil and Toni Blackholly live with their four children. When they started the programme Siannon was 12, Ceris 8, Kye 6 and Caiden just 6 months old.

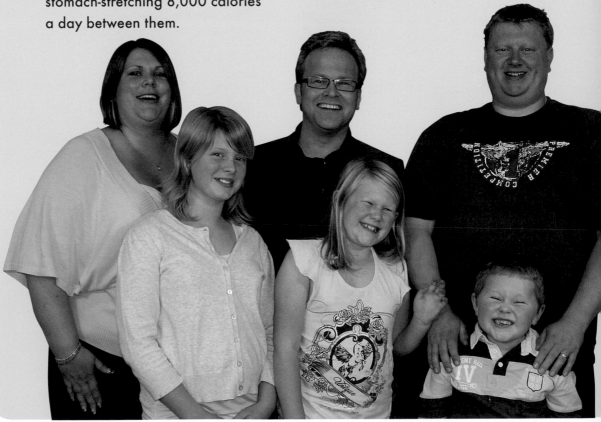

The stats
(after one year)

Dad: **Neil**
Age: **37**
Height: **5' 11"**
Start weight: **23 st 6 lb**
Now weighs: **15 st 12 lb**
Total weight loss: **7 st 8 lb**

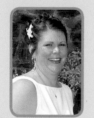

Mum: **Toni**
Age: **36**
Height: **5' 8"**
Start weight: **19 st 6 lb**
Now weighs: **14 st**
Total weight loss: **5 st 6 lb**

Total family weight loss: **13 st**

Main problem

Toni and Neil were classic junk-food addicts who never cooked anything fresh. Toni's freezer was filled with convenience foods: chicken nuggets, pizzas, pies, you name it. They ate out at fast-food chains and ordered takeaways – and the children had already begun to follow their parents' bad eating habits.

Toni knew she was feeding them the wrong foods, but was just too lazy to do anything about it.

'I hate cooking and it's convenient for me. It's there, ready-made and I just put it on a tray and stick it in the oven.'

As well as putting the children's health at risk, Neil's blood pressure was dangerously high. As a family, they did almost no exercise, even though Neil and Toni were both at home all day – Neil had been made redundant and Toni was on maternity leave from managing a petrol station.

Main motivation

With the birth of their fourth baby, Toni and Neil knew they had to do something about the way their children were growing up. They were passing on their own bad habits and the children's weight was rising – and they spent too little time exercising.

Toni and Neil are a very loving couple and Neil constantly told Toni how sexy she was. But Toni wanted to feel sexy and be able to wear the size-18 dresses she wore when they first got engaged – but she was now bursting out of size-24 clothes.

'I go to the shops and try something on and it doesn't fit so I buy the next size up. I keep thinking, what's going to happen when I run out of sizes?'

Neil: 'It makes you feel ashamed to call yourself a parent.'

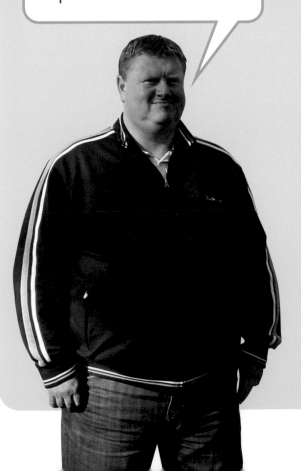

Typical day's food: Neil

Breakfast: 4 rounds of buttery toast, crisps

10am: Bacon roll and hash browns

Lunch: Sausage roll, sandwich, crisps

4pm: Sweets, kids' leftovers

7pm: Chicken curry, rice, naan and chips

9pm: Crisps, burgers

Medical tests

Obesity expert Professor David McCarthy ran tests on the Blackhollys and discovered the following:

Neil: had a dangerously high blood pressure level of 180/110, which could lead to heart disease, stroke and premature death. But he also had signs of fatty liver disease as a direct result of the very high-fat diet he was eating and this was a serious threat to his health.

Toni: was carrying the equivalent of 10 stone of fat on her body. That meant that over 50% of Toni's body weight was pure fat.

Lifestyle changes

Toni and Neil are an exceptionally loving couple who still found each other attractive but had fallen into very bad habits. Because Toni hated cooking, she found it easier to take ready meals out of the freezer and they never ate together with the children as a family.

They were very inactive and could see their children going the same way, asking for fast food and spending too much time in front of the TV.

Steve said, 'What concerns me is that, when the kids are at school, it's the perfect opportunity to do some exercise, but you just sit on your backsides on the sofa doing nothing.'

Neil had tried dieting and exercise before but always gave up and ended up putting on more weight than he'd lost so he needed a lifestyle change rather than a diet.

They needed to :

1. Learn to cook fresh food from scratch
2. Include vegetables and fruit in the whole family's diet
3. Cut out fatty snacks, such as crisps and chips
4. Involve the children in family exercise
5. Sit around the table and eat as a family

Exercise regime

Neil took up exercise like a man possessed. He joined the Nuffield House gym, where personal trainer Dawn Jolleys devised individual programmes for Neil and Toni. After checking Neil's blood pressure was normal enough to start a moderate exercise regime, she gave them an exercise plan for building up gradually to one hour of cardiovascular exercise per day.

Neil and Toni started using the home treadmill to build their cardiovascular activity. However, because Neil was competitive, within

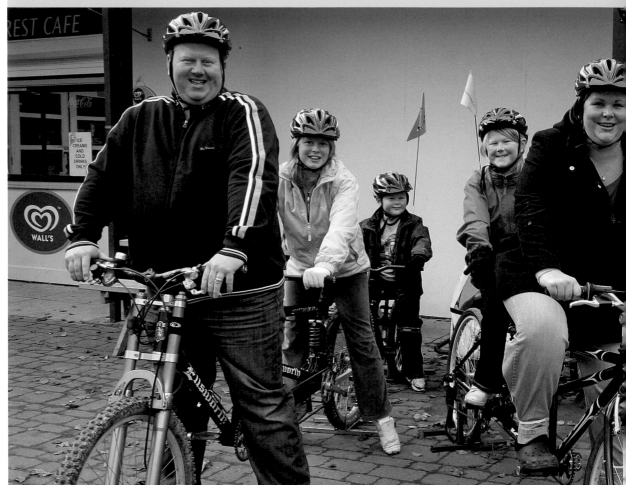

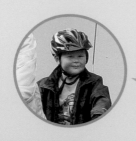

Kye: 'If Daddy gets too big, then he'll explode.'

two weeks he was running, ignoring his trainer's advice to stop. He developed a knee injury which held him back but fortunately he recovered very quickly.

Toni and Neil did circuit-based sessions based on using multiple rather than single joint actions. The aim of these sessions was to increase the calories burned and decrease the calories taken in with food so they were using more calories a day than they were taking in.

Neil and Toni were very open to any type of exercise, although Toni wasn't keen on running. However, once she was further on in her exercise programme she eagerly took up her challenge of completing a 5-mile run and proudly crossed the finish line in front of her friends and family. And now that the weight has been shed, Neil is comfortably running between 10 and 13 miles on his long runs once a week.

And the whole family is now more active, taking part in bike rides, going to the park after school and walking the dog. Neil also does classes at the gym and the whole family look and feel healthier and fitter. Even the dog!

Healthy eating

Toni had cookery lessons from Jessica Wilson, the nutritionist from the show. Uncertain of the basics, she learned how to prepare sauces rather than opt for jars and to cook healthy meals the whole family could eat together.

They threw away all the junk food from the freezer and stopped buying fizzy cola drinks, and started drinking more water. They swapped from white to wholemeal bread

immediately and started cooking casseroles full of vegetables.

The children kept a score book of what foods they liked and didn't like, although Toni learned to hide vegetables in casseroles and sauces, so they didn't always realise they were eating them.

Nutritionist Jessica Wilson said, 'Toni and Neil really needed to lead by example but with young children you have to learn what they like and then slowly introduce new tastes and textures. Eat with your children whenever possible and include them in the choices. Most children want their parents to be active and to take them to play football or go cycling and if they understand that this is the way to get more out of family life then they will come round.'

Progress highs and lows

Neil admits he was ready to quit on day 1.

'I opened the information pack from the nutritionist on what we should be eating and when, and I

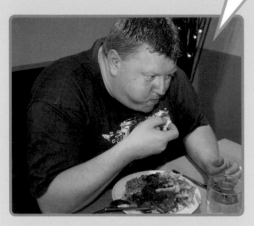

Neil: 'I could eat 15 packets of crisps on a bad day.'

found it overwhelming. There was just too much to take in in one go.

'The first couple of days were really hard going, it felt like such a change from how we had lived. I was ready to chuck it in, to be honest. But Toni kept me going, saying, let's take it one day at a time.'

Neil had another crisis when exercising so vigorously gave him knee pain and he was banned by his trainer from using the treadmill. But he did more walking under her guidance.

Converting the kids was the hard part – at first Kye wanted nothing to do with the new healthy eating plan. He wouldn't touch the fish pie and said his breakfast porridge tasted of cheesy feet! It took some time but by staying strong and leading by example Toni and Neil won the day.

The family says:

Neil: 'Being told about my health problems was like being hit with a brick – it was a real wake-up call. And I could see what we were doing to the children. This isn't a diet, it's a change of life and we couldn't have done it without each other.

'We used to collect the kids from school and make excuses not to go to the park – now they play there every day and we walk the dog around it.

'I have so much more confidence – I got a new job and I don't think I would have got it without this. I look so much better – I used to have dry skin on my elbows and knees and now that's cleared up.

'I once weighed myself with Ceris on my back and I still weighed less than when I started and I realised that I was carrying around a whole other person. Toni and I joke that between us we've lost a whole Steve Miller!

'I didn't understand about what was in food before, but since I started choosing healthy food I no longer crave bags of crisps – I find it hard to believe I used to eat 15 packs a day.

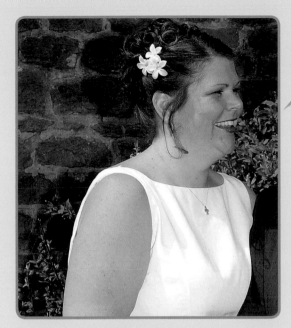

Toni: 'I can't wait to go on holiday because I'm going to wear a bikini.'

'And the children naturally eat more healthily – their school lunch boxes have wholemeal sandwiches or wraps, nuts, yoghurt and fruit, and they don't come home starving hungry. And Kye used to be so hyperactive and now his behaviour is much calmer.'

Toni: 'It's made an incredible difference. I have energy to play with the children. We walk the dog, they have a trampoline, a swing and ride their bikes. I get such a boost out of shopping for clothes in normal shops and although Neil always used to tell me I looked sexy, I can now look at myself in the mirror and think, "Yes, you do look good."

'People think you can't enjoy food any more but you can – you just eat in a controlled way. We can still go for a curry or go to parties, you are just aware of what you are eating. I've lost the taste for a lot of things – I can pass a chip shop or burger van and just smell the grease.

'And I've learned to cook! If the kids want a pizza as a treat I make it with home-made sauce instead of stuff from a jar. They don't keep asking for rubbish any more, they eat muesli and porridge, and brown rice and apples – things they wouldn't have touched before.'

The Blackholly family's top tips

- Find your motivation. Try buying something in a size too small and really work to fit into it.

- Stay positive even if you have a bad week and only lose a pound – it's still better than nothing.

- Get help and support – it's easier to work together than on your own.

- Never skip breakfast.

- Understand food values – don't assume some things are healthy and some not, do your homework.
- If you haven't got a dog, borrow one – a daily walk in the park is great exercise and the kids love it too.

Inconvenience truths!

With four young children it's not surprising that Toni sometimes feels too exhausted to cook meals, but the truth is that many healthy meals take less time to cook than throwing chicken nuggets and chips in the oven. And you can even have a delicious healthy version of chicken and chips, just not coated in fatty batter or crumbs.

And using prepared foods means you have no idea what's actually in them. Take a breakfast of puffed rice cereal with milk, for example.

- 1 small 60 g portion of puffed rice cereal with milk every day for a year = 6.5 kg of sugar
- 1 small 60 g portion of chocolate puffed rice with milk every day for a year = 11.6 kg of sugar

And that's not counting the sugar you might sprinkle on top!

Whereas a bowl of porridge made with water contains the equivalent of just ¼ teaspoon of sugar – that's just 0.38 kg over the course of a year.

Neil's 15 packets of crisps a day alone meant that he was consuming over 70 litres of vegetable oil over a year. Even eating just one packet of crisps a day equates to downing neary 5 litres of vegetable oil a year!

What else are you eating when you eat fast food? Remember that fast food and convenience food have many other things added to them that can affect your daily intake of calories and sodium, such as sugar, fat and excess salt.

So although Chicken McNuggets claim to be made with 100% breast meat, the meat actually makes up less than half the nugget (45%, according to McDonald's website). The rest is a combination of batter, flavour enhancers, oils and other ingredients.

Coating strips of breast meat at home with egg and breadcrumbs means you know exactly what you're putting into your children's mouths.

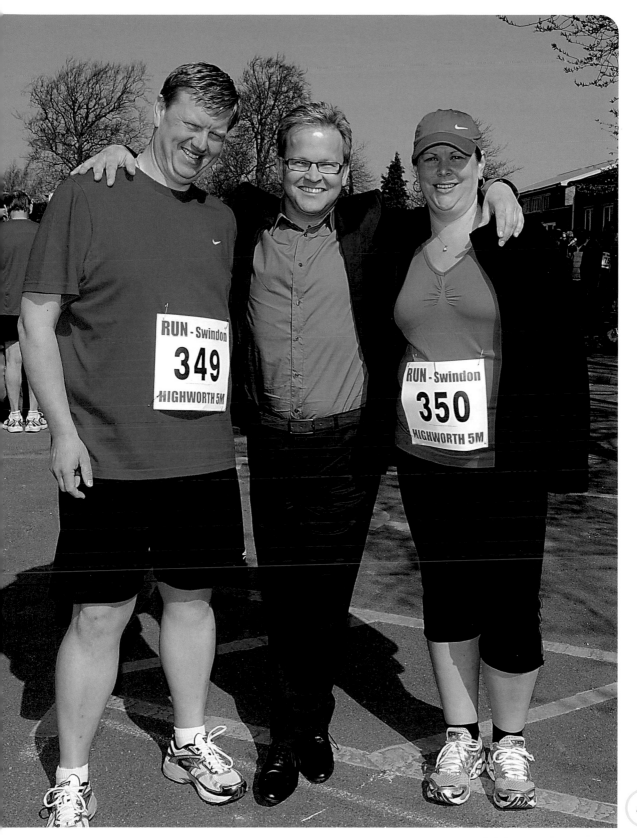

RUN - Swindon
349
HIGHWORTH 5M

RUN - Swindon
350
HIGHWORTH 5M

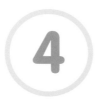

Motivation

Why do you want to lose weight and get fit? Perhaps you want to look more attractive, or you're anxious about the health risks of being overweight, or you're worried that your children are following in your footsteps and piling on the pounds. It's probably a mixture of all these reasons, but whatever drove you to pick up this book is the same reason that will help you to achieve your aim of living a healthier life; one that will make you slimmer, fitter and more confident.

Personal motivation is a powerful force that you can harness and use to drive yourself forward out of the fat habits that are holding you back.

No one knows more about motivation than *Fat Families* presenter Steve Miller, who runs a training and motivation company – and, more importantly, is a former member of the Fat Club himself! He advises people trying to lose weight to focus on the real reason why they are doing it and to set themselves goals, things they really want to achieve in their new slimmer, fit life.

> 'If you haven't got an ounce of motivation, you won't lose an ounce of fat.' Steve

It's as simple as that. Losing weight and getting fit is all about attitude, and unless you find a good reason for changing your family's life, you won't stick to it.

It's no good other people telling you to do it, you have to know and believe that your life will be better if there's less of you. And you need to be honest with yourself. We all know that being fat has huge health risks and if you ask an overweight person if they want to lose weight for their health they'll almost certainly say yes. But what really motivates most people is that they want to look and feel better about themselves. They want to feel more confident, they want better self-esteem and they want to be able to buy clothes in high-street shops instead of having to shop online for outsize versions.

So what's stopping us shedding those pounds? Excuses! Which is where tough-talking Steve Miller comes in.

WEIGHT LOSS AIMS
An average weight loss is 2 lb a week, but very obese people should aim for more than that, and as they get lighter it will tail off.

Steve used to be fat and knows all about making excuses – he made them for long enough himself. It's hard to make the decision to stop being fat but that's what it is – a decision, and too many people don't want to make it. Steve's tough-talking method puts the responsibility firmly back on you. He has no time for people who blame other causes and don't take responsibility for themselves. It's become commonplace for overweight people to blame food manufacturers and even the government for the fact they're fat and unfit.

Well, if the government hasn't got it through to you yet that you should be eating five portions of fruit and vegetables a day, you must be living in a cave. Most people know exactly what they should be eating and what makes them fat, but they carry on eating the wrong things – and in massive amounts.

Steve admits that when he was fat his confidence was low, and he would go out and think everyone was looking at his partner and wondering why on earth he was with Steve. One day, he says, he was aware of people mocking and mimicking him for being fat and he went home and decided, 'That's it. Enough.' He took the decision to change his life and never turned back.

When Steve was working with the Huzzey family, daughter Kayleigh got really angry with him for printing mugs and place mats with pictures on them of how fat she might end up. Steve was thrilled – it meant she cared about what he was saying. She was bothered and wanted to prove him wrong, which motivated her to change.

So you have to change your attitude to eating, exercise and your entire lifestyle, and to do that you have to have some motivation.

'I'm not always popular with the people I work with because I tell it like it is!' Steve

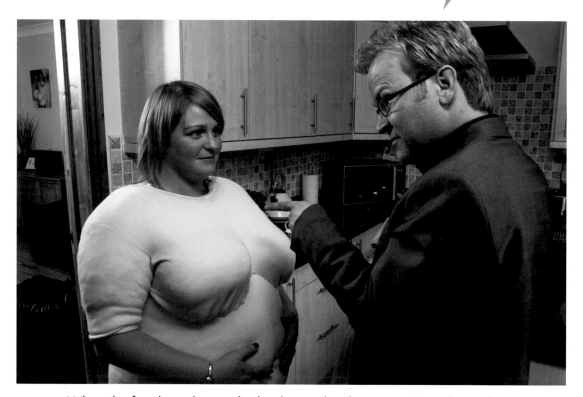

When the families who applied to be on the show meet Steve he makes them confront some truths about themselves that they don't like. He makes them see themselves physically as other people see them. He spells out the damage they're doing to their bodies. And not just theirs, but other people's in the family, because most families eat in the same way. And if you make yourself ill through bad habits, it doesn't just affect you, it affects the people who love you.

But you need to trust in someone who will tell you the truth – and then encourage you to change (see his tip on 'Radiators, not Drains' on page 53).

And then you have to really want to change, not just for a few weeks or months – that's called a diet and you won't keep it up. You have to shed your old life like a skin and step out of it prepared to become a different person. Which is why taking the challenge as a family or a couple is a great way to motivate other people and take strength from their support.

Everyone has a good reason to stop being fat and to take more exercise. You just need to stop hiding behind the comfort of a kebab and find what your personal motivation is. Here are some tips from Steve himself to help keep going.

Steve's top ten motivation tips

1. No excuses!

There are no excuses. I've heard them all and, believe me, none of them are worth anything. They're holding you back. Here are a few common excuses and why they're not good enough.

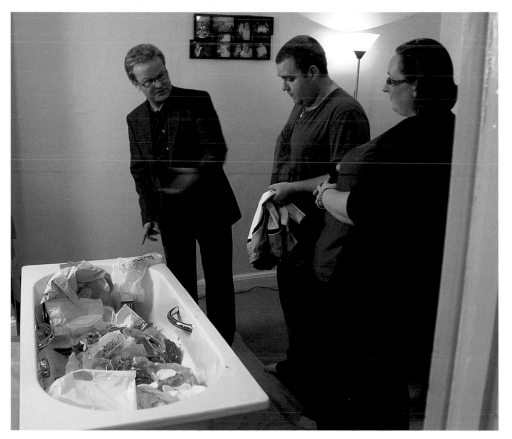

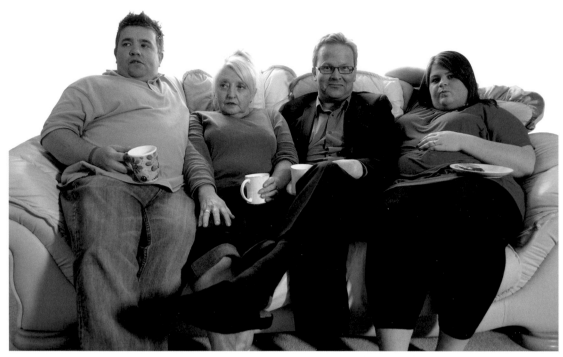

'We haven't got time' to do exercise, plan meals in advance, shop healthily.

Who hasn't got time to walk up a few flights of stairs instead of using the lift? I see people waiting for lifts to go up a couple of floors and in the time they are waiting they could have walked up the stairs. You've got time to watch TV so you've got time to chop a few vegetables and do a stir-fry instead of wolfing down a pizza. We're all busy but if you want to lose weight you'll make time.

> **FACT**
> **An obese person dies on average nine years earlier than someone of normal weight.**

'I hardly eat anything, I don't know why I put on weight.'

That's scientifically impossible – unless you have a rare medical condition. Doctors fall about laughing at this one. You're fat because you eat too much of the wrong food and you don't work it off. If you think you don't eat much, keep a food diary and write down everything you eat and drink – and I mean everything, not just main meals. All those milky coffees, chocolate biscuits, bags of crisps. Just because you eat on the run doesn't mean the food doesn't have calories. Write it down for a week, then say you don't eat anything ...

'It's too expensive to eat healthily.'

I've done a shopping price comparison and it simply isn't true that you can't eat healthily on a budget (see pages 62–63 for an example). Go to a market or even a supermarket at the very end of the day and see what fresh-food bargains you can get. Cook up a vegetable soup and see what that works out as per portion. Then add up the money you spend on takeaways. Also there's a knock-on effect to being fat – think how much more you spend on clothes from outsize shops, for instance.

'It's not my fault, it's the food industry's fault for making such sweet, fatty foods.'

Well, you don't have to eat them! They only make them because you buy them. Take responsibility for what you put in your own mouth. The supermarket might be full of rubbishy food but it's also full of fruit, vegetables, lean meat, fish – there's never been more choice of healthy foods to eat but if you walk past them straight to the pizza fridge that's your choice. Plenty of other people walk past the pizzas to the fresh vegetable stand – why not follow them for a change?

'I can't afford to go to the gym.'

Then don't go. I don't, but I walk, all the time. If you can't afford a gym you can walk for nothing, anywhere, any time. People whinge to me that there isn't a park nearby (excuse, excuse) – so walk on the pavements, it's what they're for. Thousands of runners pound the pavements every day, so you can walk around your local area without people thinking you're weird! Use all the strategies in this book about how to up your intensity level.

Walk an extra stop if you take the bus to work and walk to the shops. If the kids' school really is a long way away and you have to drive (how did kids get to school before we all had cars?!), then park the car ten minutes' walk from school and you can all walk that last bit. I know we're all rushed in the morning but get up ten minutes earlier – do you really want to lose weight or not?

Dave Turner works incredibly long hours but now gets up an hour earlier every day to walk on his treadmill – and he walks home from work. Then he and his wife Keri go for long walks along the cliffs of Barry. And if you want to see the astonishing transformation it's made to his health, just turn to page 194.

Lots of towns have walking clubs if you don't like the idea of walking on your own – look them up on the internet and see if there's one local to you.

Buy a skipping rope – it won't break the bank – if heavyweight boxers can learn to skip, then so can you!

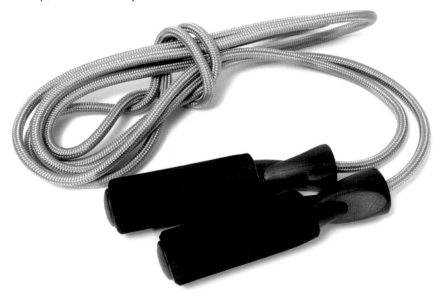

Write down a list of all the excuses you use for being fat and unfit (they're not reasons, remember, they're excuses) and make a conscious decision to let them all go by tearing the list up.

2. Draw a picture of your ideal body shape

And keep it on you at all times. Most overweight people don't want to look at themselves – I notice that some overweight families don't actually have a full-length mirror in their homes. But confronting the truth about what you look like is one of the main motivators for losing weight. When we use the tiny camera to look in close-up at our fat familes' bodies, they are genuinely shocked at what they see – they might use a face mirror to shave or put on make-up but they don't look at the state of their bellies and bottoms.

So keep with you all the time a target of what you aim to look like and it will reinforce why you are doing this. Once the weight starts to drop off – and it will – you'll need to do some exercise to tone yourself up. You don't want to hang on to that old body, you want to carve yourself a new one that you can dress in different clothes and show off! Having a visual reminder of where you are heading is a powerful motivator.

3. Hang up an item of clothing two sizes smaller

There's not an overweight person in the world who hasn't got an outfit in the wardrobe that's two sizes too small – but that person keeps it in the hope that they 'might fit back into it'. This doesn't just apply to women, there are plenty of men out there with jackets and trousers at the back of the wardrobe that haven't

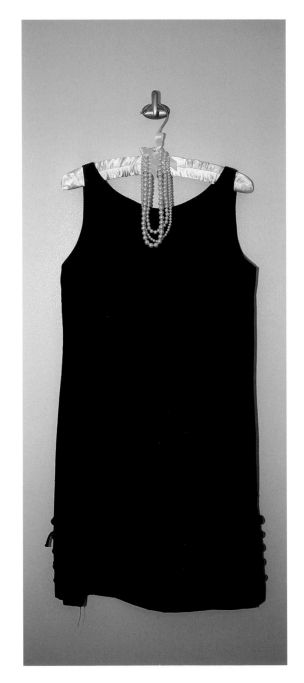

had an outing for a good few years. Well, get it out because its time has come. Or buy yourself something new you really like in a size you aim to become. Hang it up where you can see it every day – in the dining room to remind you to eat less, or near the TV to remind you to get off your bum and do something.

It's better still if the outfit has special happy memories attached to it, like Toni Blackholly's engagement dress (see page 59), so that you have an emotional association too.

This is your carrot – and once you're in the swing of changing your body shape, you'll find that fitting into this isn't an end in itself, it's just a step on the ladder of what you can achieve.

4. Get a weight-loss family charter board

Get the whole family to work out a set of ideals and write them on a charter board. Write down the agreed routine, e.g. swimming on Tuesday, an hour's walk on Sunday, etc. so no one can pretend they forgot. Write down the ways in which you are going to change the family's eating habits – fresh fruit for dessert, no sugar in teas, breakfast every single day, etc. This is your life-change plan and it needs to be open, honest and with no room for misunderstanding – deliberate or otherwise!

Record your weight loss every week. Men often like the competitive element of this. This is fine if that motivates you but remember you are supporting each other, not trying to do each other down. If someone's weight loss stalls one week, you'll all be able to see this on the chart and offer a bit of encouragement or look back over the week and see why they've levelled off. Did they pig out at a party? Were they a bit under the weather so didn't exercise? Perhaps they've reached a plateau and need to be doing a bit more exercise, or increasing the intensity. Act as a team and don't make someone feel isolated. It might be you next week …

5. Surround yourself with Radiators, not Drains

Don't listen to **Drains** – people who are negative about what you're doing. Some 'friends' will try to persuade you that you don't really need to lose weight, that you're not so much fun now that you're not knocking back the booze and burgers. They are trying to drain your energy. Drains keep you fat.

You need **Radiators**, who will be positive and encouraging, will cheer you on for every pound you lose and actively help you to change your lifestyle. Remember, this is all about attitude and you don't need people who play mind games.

Beware of the partner or friend who is a little jealous that you're succeeding and starts 'feeding' you on the quiet. They might suggest a bit of ice cream and give you a bigger portion, or start buying in snacks when you've agreed not to have them in the house. (At times like these, remember the charter board.)

As a family you need to agree there will be no game playing. The Huzzeys were an extraordinarily straightforward and supportive family – no mind games and everyone lost tons of weight (well, not literally tons, but almost!).

But don't expect your Radiators to provide sympathy if you fall back on old excuses. Radiators are warm and understanding but they're not there to molly-coddle you. The nourishment they provide should be emotional, not comfort food.

6. Develop affirmations and chant them

Start thinking about the way you talk about food and exercise, and see how loaded your words are. This is especially important if you have children. Do you say, 'I'm going to be good today and not eat chocolate'? Why load eating with negative thoughts and guilt? Why divide behaviour into good and bad?

Wake up and say, 'I'm going to enjoy what I'm eating today.' Don't be afraid of food or see it as something you have to fight against.

Jan Huzzey says, 'I'm the gov'nor now,' which is a brilliant way of describing the fact that she controls her eating rather than it controlling her.

Don't keep telling your children that eating this food is healthy, but eating that one is bad, or they'll develop an emotionally confused relationship with food. If you just feed them healthily without making a big thing of it they'll develop healthy habits. Food choices should become unconscious – you reach for an apple for a snack not a biscuit because that's your way of life.

Develop a few positive affirmations you can chant to yourself every day and they will keep you strong and positive. Try: 'I'm looking forward to walking to work', 'I can't wait to get to the gym', 'I'm in charge of what I eat,' or 'I have more energy when I eat healthy food.'

7. Walk tall

From the first day you start your new life you should pull yourself up and walk tall. Many fat people try to hide themselves by looking down and shrinking away from eye contact. But you are now losing weight so you need to be positive about the new you and be confident. Steve Joell-Ireland goes swimming at his local pool and feels on top of the world because inside he knows he has ditched the fat Steve and is confident in his new self – and he doesn't care how other people look at him.

Walking tall works on two levels – it literally makes you carry yourself better, but it's more about building your inner confidence and taking part in the life around you. You deserve to be noticed because you are achieving something positive. Your self-esteem is improving from day one because you have taken a life-changing decision. Other people respond to confidence and the more you put out there, the more you'll get back.

8. Look at fat people's behaviour

People are always very shocked when I say this but it really works as a motivational technique. I know it's not politically correct but if you want tissues and sympathy because you're fat, you've come to the wrong person!

Stand outside the chip shop or burger bar and see how many people buying fish and chips are overweight. Sit in a café and look at the fat people eating knickerbocker glories or sausage and chips. They claim they have the right to eat what they want – and they have – but you have the right not to be like that. You can turn your back on that behaviour once you see how absurd it is. Watch how quickly they eat – it's like a famine is on the way – because they're not tasting and enjoying the flavour of that food. They may even be eating it as a comfort because they are unhappy being fat. Recognise your old self and feel proud that you're not like that now. Watch them walking really slowly because they're out of breath. Watch them spill over onto your seat in an aeroplane or on a bus. All these things are avoidable and reversible.

But don't think that because you are changing your life around that you can never have a cake or an ice cream again. Some of the fat families I work with think I've lived a really deprived life! They say to me, 'I bet you never have a cake, Steve.' I do, of course, but it's a conscious decision, not a habit. And often people don't actually want a whole cake, just a couple of bites to taste the sweetness, so why not have one between two of you when you're out for a coffee – you really won't feel the need to scoff a whole one.

Once you've changed your mind-set and realised that you are in control, you will be able to make small changes all the time, and all those small changes add up to lost pounds.

9. Don't overload your plate

Just because it's there, you don't have to finish it! Stop feeling guilty. Maybe you were brought up by parents who said, 'Eat everything you're given, starving children in Africa would be glad of that.' But although it is terrible how much food we waste, shovelling down every last roast potato you've loaded onto your plate isn't the answer. If you hadn't cooked so many, there wouldn't be anything to waste ...

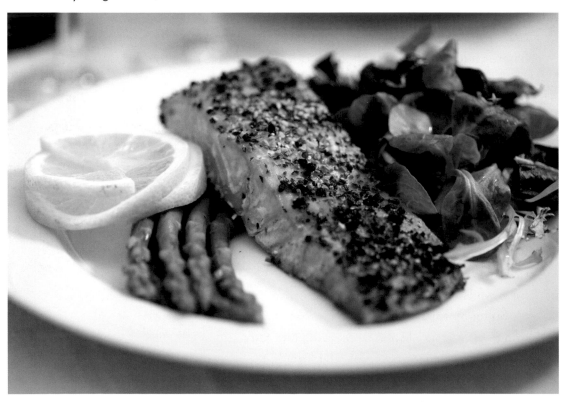

Watch people at a buffet table piling so much food on their plates they can hardly balance it – as if this is their last meal for a month. Take a small portion, and see if that satisfies you. Once you get in the habit of knowing the right portion size, you'll stop overloading your plate.

Leaving something on the plate empowers you – you have made the choice not to eat the last bit because you have control and know that you don't need it.

If you're really worried about the children in Africa, give some money to charity – that will do them more good than you getting fatter.

10. Reward yourself

Motivation is about giving yourself reasons to change, so when you achieve something, whether that's a certain weight loss, or meeting a fitness challenge, or getting into that special dress or pair of trousers, reward yourself. Just don't use food as a reward!

Buy yourself a bright, cheerful bunch of flowers, or some new make-up or a DVD, or go to the cinema. You don't even have to spend money – run yourself an indulgent, foamy bath and relax with a book or meet up with some friends you haven't seen for a while.

So many families make the mistake of using sugary fatty foods as rewards and they pass this mentality on to their children. 'Eat your vegetables and you can have some ice cream,' means to a child, 'Vegetables are horrible so I'm bribing you to eat them. Ice cream is lovely and you get it for being good.' And what attitudes to food will they grow up with?

Rewards are a great way of motivating yourself too – reach a target, take your reward, set a new target. Even when you've reached your absolute desired weight you can still have targets in life – keeping it off, for a start! But use your new-found confidence to challenge yourself in other areas – maybe apply for a better job or study for an exam or take up a new hobby. You've left the old you behind and there's no limit to what the new you can do.

Aversion technique

One of the techniques Steve uses to motivate people to ditch the junk is aversion therapy, and you can do this yourself.

Basically, you learn to associate something you want to give up – sweet, fatty foods, for example – with something really horrible, that literally makes you feel sick. Everyone has different revulsion points – the more extreme, the better!

Eileen Haddrell really hates jellied eels and cottage cheese. So Steve took her to a restaurant, ordered her a favourite chocolate dessert and made her close her eyes and imagine it covered in slimy, slippery jellied eels and creamy lumps of cottage cheese. She had to picture those things on the chocolate, on the spoon she would use to eat it, the whole thing. Then she had to open her eyes and imagine it while looking at the chocolate – and then they did it for real. Poor Eileen nearly threw up! But it worked and she can now picture that when she sees a tempting chocolate dessert – and she can say, 'No thanks!' pretty quickly …

Stephen and James Joell-Ireland needed to be weaned off pizzas so Steve ordered a big cheesy, doughy pizza and mashed it all up in a bowl with loads of oil, all the oil that would be used to make it. He made them dip their fingers in the oily mush, smell it and then drink some of that greasy fat – after all, that's what they are putting in their stomachs. Surprisingly, the pizza didn't seem so appealing when they imagined it in that state! Simple but effective.

With Toni and Neil Blackholly, who loved their takeaway food, the trick was to order their favourite Indian dish, liquidise it and put it in a glass jar. Every day they had to get it out of the cupboard, open the jar and smell it as it started to go off – it was really disgusting – but that's exactly what they were putting in their stomachs a few times a week. Toni was appalled by the technique but, again, shock tactics are the ones that stick.

Try it with your own weak areas – really go to town with the most disgusting combination of vomit-inducing ingredients you can think of. They don't have to be food – imagine mice droppings or whatever gives you the shivers all over that ham and cheese-filled croissant. Mmm ...

Motivation targets

Each of the families from the show needed something special to motivate them – apart from general health concerns and wanting to look and feel better. So they were given a visible target that they could have as a reminder of why they were running on the treadmill or dumping the junk.

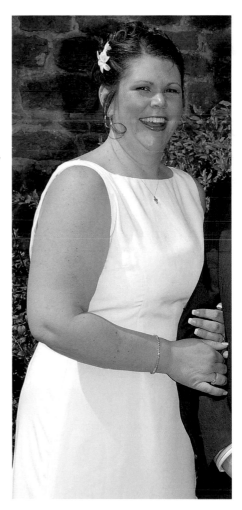

Toni Blackholly (right) was desperate to fit back into the dress she wore when she and Neil got engaged, so she hung it up on the wall. At the beginning of the healthy-living change she was wearing a size 24, and the dress was a size 18, so she had some way to go. It was a real incentive and when the pounds started to melt and she discovered she did have a waist after all, that dress became a possibility. Now, of course, it's far too big and she's fitting into size 14s. But the dress did what it was supposed to do and now it's back in the wardrobe for the right reason!

Jan Huzzey (below) is a real glamour girl now she's ditched the booze and buns. She was tempted by a sexy pair of high heels that her chubby feet couldn't squeeze into – and she was so determined to shed her frumpy image that she now looks like a totally different person.

Phil Huzzey (right), of course, had his major health problems hanging over him as a reminder of why he had to lose weight.

Sadie Turner (see page 194) was a young woman who wanted to dress for her age, but her size was stopping her. Living near the beach, she really

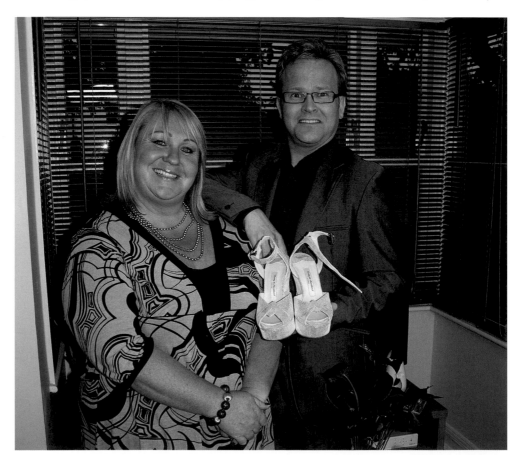

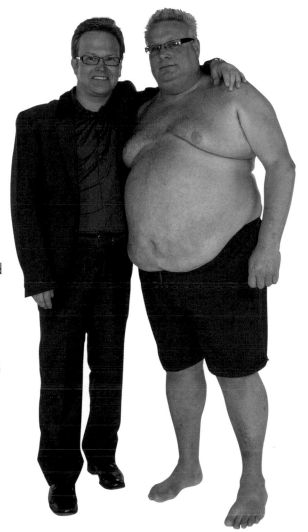

wanted to be able to wear a size-14 bikini instead of the size 20 that she currently wore. To help motivate her weight loss, Steve bought her a beautiful dress that was two sizes too small and hung it up so she could see it every day. It really worked – well, for a while, at least. Now it's too big!

Linda Haddrell (see page 114) was swallowing loads of tablets every day for her weight-related health problems and really wanted to get fit to improve her energy levels. She was open and honest about what she found hard but was a real fighter and now she has been able, under guidance from her doctor, to come off almost all her medication. That is a real change of lifestyle and she says she now feels 40 instead of nearly 60. If ever there was a story to inspire others, it's being able to come off medication through your own efforts.

Matthew and Sarah (see page 115) from the Haddrell family wanted to start a family but were worried that their weight would make it difficult for Sarah to conceive. And as fat, unfit parents, they worried that they would be bad role models for their future children. They were given some little baby clothes to hang up on the wall to remind them that this was why they were making the changes. The weight has just melted away.

Find your own motivational target to keep you on the straight and narrow. Whether it's a health- or size-related target, if you have a fixed goal to strive for you're much more likely to stay on your new healthy regime.

Save money with healthy food

Eating well doesn't have to cost a lot of money. This shopping list was done for the Brookes in series two of the show. It provides food for three days for two adults and comes to just £20.94 in total*. That's £6.98 per day – only £3.49 per adult per day! So saving money can be part of your motivation for eating healthily.

Day 1

Breakfast: Egg on toast with mushrooms and tomato (for 2)

Lunch: Jacket potato with beans (for 2)

Dinner: Vegetable chilli with brown rice (for 2)

Day 2

Breakfast: Porridge with banana (for 2)

Lunch: Wholemeal bread sandwiches with chicken and salad/ egg mayonnaise and salad (for 2)

Dinner: Chicken stir-fry

Day 3

Breakfast: Beans on toast/ Bacon sandwich

Lunch: Greek salad (for 2)

Dinner: Tuna pasta (for 2)

Snacks

8 bananas

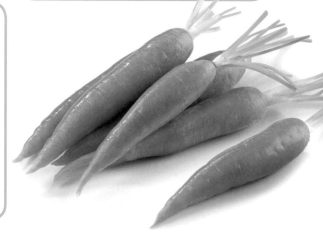

Shopping basket

Product	Quantity	Price
Water (2 litres)	x 3	£0.54
Vegetable stir-fry (650 g)	x 1	£1.00
Bananas	x 8	£1.00
Chicken breast (300 g)	x 1	£2.50
Semi-skimmed milk (568 ml/1 pint)	x 1	£0.45
Morinaga firm tofu (349 g)	x 1	£1.00
Tuna chunks (185 g)	x 1	£0.55
Sweetcorn in water (198 g)	x 1	£0.20
Spaghetti (500 g)	x 1	£0.39
Low-fat Greek-style cheese (200 g)	x 1	£1.50
Beans in tomato sauce (420 g)	x 2	£0.58
Unsmoked bacon (300 g)	x 1	£1.46
Instant hot oat cereal (500 g)	x 1	£0.75
Muesli (1 kg)	x 1	£0.65

Product	Quantity	Price
Red kidney beans in water (420 g)	x 1	£0.19
Carrots (1 kg)	x 1	£0.75
Peppers (600 g)	x 1	£1.25
Garlic	x 1	£0.25
Onions	x 2	£0.27
Iceberg lettuce	x 1	£0.55
Potatoes (2.5 kg)	x 1	£0.99
Chopped tomatoes (400 g)	x 2	£0.66
Tomatoes (450 g)	x 1	£0.74
Mushrooms (400 g)	x 1	£0.89
Barn eggs (box of 6)	x 1	£0.63
Medium wholemeal loaf (800 g)	x 1	£0.47
Sweet potatoes	x 2	£0.54
Courgettes	x 1	£0.19

Total: £20.94

*Please note that these prices are correct for a shopping basket from Sainsburys in August 2010.

Motivation

The Huzzey family from Essex

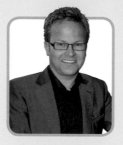

Steve visited the Huzzeys from Essex.

'Life for the Huzzeys had been one long party ... until the calories and cholesterol finally caught up with Phil and he suffered a double heart attack.

'Weight loss for this family was literally a matter of life or death but their biggest weaknesses were big oily curries ... and booze. Jan and Phil had been drinking more than five times the recommended daily limit. So with eating and drinking like there's no tomorrow between them, the three of them were gulping down 11,500 calories a day!'

The stats (after one year)

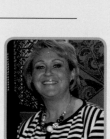

Dad: **Phil**
Age: **45**
Height: **5' 9"**
Start weight: **22 st 4 lb**
Now weighs: **15 st 12 lb**

Total weight loss: **6 st 6 lb**

Mum: **Jan**
Age: **45**
Height: **5' 2"**
Start weight: **19 st**
Now weighs: **12 st**

Total weight loss: **7 st**

Daughter: **Kayleigh**
Age: **24**
Height: **5' 3"**
Start weight: **14 st 7 lb**
Now weighs: **11 st 10 lb**

Total weight loss: **2 st 11 lb**

Total family weight loss: 16 st 3 lb

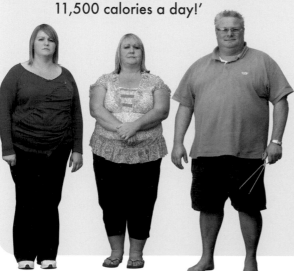

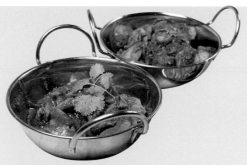

Main problem

Phil had recently had a heart attack and his lifestyle was partly to blame.

The family enjoyed the party life with lots of socialising. Family dinners were built around huge meals and lots of booze! They had returned from living in Spain, where they had piled on the pounds eating paella and enjoying the local wines. They did little exercise and had given up quickly on previous diets, so the weight piled back on.

One of the Huzzeys' weaknesses was curry – takeaway and home-made. When they cooked at home they used enough oil to make a curry for 15 people! A curry for four needs only about two tablespoons of oil.

Since his heart attack, Phil, a fishing guide, was at home all day and spent most of his time sitting in front of the television. Kayleigh worked four days a week and had a baby so did no exercise and ate huge meals. She wasn't a snacker but loved her rich sauces and curries.

Main motivation

Phil and his family were terrified he might have another heart attack. Obesity runs in his family: his father was over 26 stone when he died and his grandfather even heavier. Jan's family is also overweight; her brother had weight-loss surgery. Phil's heart attack was a wake-up call and the family wanted to regain their health.

Kayleigh wanted to be part of the team, helping her dad as well as losing weight for herself. She hoped appearing on TV would give her the incentive to keep going.

Typical day's food: Jan

Breakfast:	Fry-up bacon sandwich: 2 slices of bread, 3 slices of bacon, fried mushrooms
11am:	Snack of five biscuits
Lunch:	2 ham rolls, packet of crisps, cake or chocolate bar
4pm:	Biscuits and crisps
6pm:	Takeaway Indian: curry, pilau rice, roast potatoes, naan, poppadoms
9pm:	Snacks, sandwich, cakes or doughnuts, several glasses of wine (more on weekends)

The Huzzey family

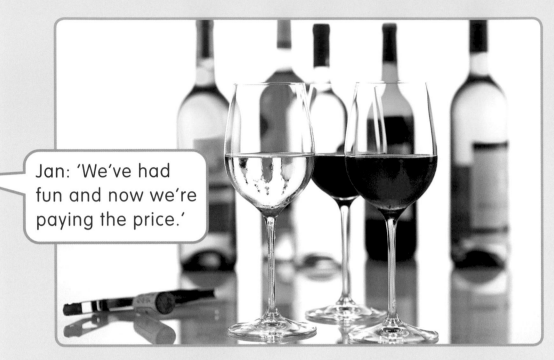

Jan: 'We've had fun and now we're paying the price.'

Alcohol: Jan and Phil had been drinking more than five times the recommended daily limit.

Their weekly combined intake of booze was around:

12 bottles of wine

10 pints of lager

1 pint of brandy

1 pint of vodka

That's around 10,200 calories per week!

Medical tests

We ran tests on the Huzzeys and discovered that:

Phil: had abnormal liver function, which could be a result of his alcohol intake or part of another illness called Metabolic Syndrome. Phil displayed all the symptoms of Metabolic Syndrome, which included abdominal obesity, high blood pressure and high cholesterol.

And when you've already had a heart attack, this is just adding to the risk of another one. Phil's current weight was life-threatening.

Jan: Jan's tests were better but, alarmingly, over 52% of Jan's body was fat. She needed to shed some pounds, fast.

Kayleigh: Like her Dad, Kayleigh had high cholesterol – even though she was just 24 there was a chance she could have done some damage to her heart already.

Lifestyle changes

The Huzzeys are a fun, happy family who believe in living life to the full – they love entertaining family and friends, hearty curries and a drink – or six.

But the reality of Phil's heart attack scared them all. They realised that Phil was still drinking and eating way more than he should have been.

The Huzzeys needed to change their lives quickly. They could still socialise and have family meals but they needed to:

1. Cut back on the booze
2. Cut back on the size of their meals
3. Cut back on the oil and fat in their home-cooked meals and takeaways
4. Start exercising as a family

Jan: 'Sometimes I could really cry for Kayleigh because I know exactly what she's going through and I'd hate her to live her life the way I've had to live mine.'

Exercise regime

Personal trainer Russell Byham took on the Huzzeys with a brief to get them moving and shift some weight quickly.

As Phil had already had a heart attack and Jan had admitted she hated any form of exercise, Russell knew he had a big job on his hands!

'At the beginning they could hardly walk up the stairs without getting out of breath, so any increase in activity was going to show an improvement quite quickly.

'With Phil we had to ease him into it because of his heart problems. The programme was very gentle to begin with and Phil wore a heart-rate

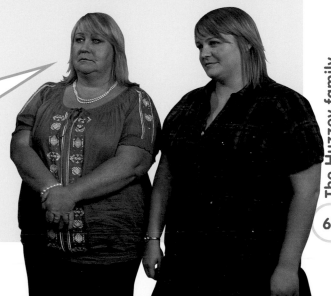

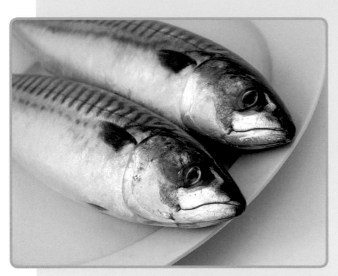

monitor so we could see exactly what his heart was up to.

'Basically we started by getting them to walk – they'd had a very lazy lifestyle in Spain so just walking to places or in the park was a start. There's no point throwing people in the deep end – and most importantly they've got to discover what they like doing.

'They even tried some dance lessons – and dance is a great exercise, especially for teenagers.

'Kayleigh hit a bit of a plateau with exercise and I knew we had to find something she would enjoy or she'd lose interest – so we got her boxing.

She loved it – all kitted out in the gloves and pads – she really wanted to do it. It was totally different from what we were doing with Phil and Jan because we tried to stay away from upper-body exercise with Phil so as not to put a strain on his heart. After about three or four weeks we introduced a bit of circuit training with squats and stability boards. Jan was keen to do something together with Phil; it can be quite intimidating when a fitness trainer turns up and we needed to make her laugh and feel at ease.

'You have to use a bit of psychology, make them want to achieve but also find out what they enjoy so they'll rise to the challenge.

'They lost a lot of weight quickly so we could afford to up their level of activity by about 5% each time. At

Phil: 'I can't afford to have another heart attack. I'm concerned about my children and my wife, leaving them and causing them grief for the rest of their lives.'

the beginning of the programme we could only do about half an hour a day and I'd spend time explaining exactly what was happening to their bodies when they exercised and how much you need to do to burn off the sort of food they had been eating.

'Sometimes the actual weight loss can slow a bit but if you keep measuring the body you see that the inches are coming off and the muscle mass is building. And as the Huzzeys increased their percentage of lean muscle, that was burning more fat.

'I think they should be really proud of what they've achieved.'

Phil admitted, 'It can be hard at the beginning – Jan hates exercise and hated the treadmill so we went for walks instead. It was good for us because it meant we talked more – when you're sitting in front of the TV or computer you don't talk to one another.'

Healthy eating

Expert nutritionist Jessica Wilson was concerned that Phil's diet needed to reflect that he had heart problems so wanted to up the amount of omega-3 oils he ate. Omega-3 oils are found in oily fish such as mackerel and salmon, and few people eat anywhere near enough.

Magnesium is thought to be good for heart problems so Jessica upped the level of green leafy vegetables and whole grains, and encouraged the use of garlic and onion.

'Like all the families I work with, the Huzzeys ate too much – and drank too much – but they were so determined to turn things around that they really took the advice on board. The Huzzeys were great entertainers but the problem with that lifestyle is that when you're having a good time you don't notice how much you're drinking – and liquid calories are no different to solid ones. Never mind all the other damage booze does.

Steve: 'The furthest these guys used to wobble was from the sofa to the fridge. Now there's no stopping them.'

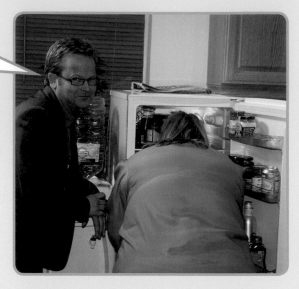

'But by cooking home-made curries with less oil they could still eat their favourite foods, just more healthily. You don't have to stop partying, you just do it more healthily. If you look at the family now, they're transformed but they're still having fun!'

Progress highs and lows

In the first week Jan lost 8 lb, Phil lost 7 lb and Kayleigh lost 2 lb.

Kayleigh, who has a young baby, started to struggle with fitting exercise into her daily routine and her weight loss slowed down to just a pound a week.

Steve advised her to meet up with Mum and Dad every day to exercise with them – after the first five or six weeks, many people struggle to keep going and the temptation is to give up, but the more you work as a family, the less likely you are to give up.

Steve also dressed Kayleigh up in a fat suit that was the same size and weight as her mum to make her realise where she'd end up if she didn't put in the effort. And he gave her pictures of herself to motivate her. All this made her determined to prove him wrong about being lazy, so she climbed back on board.

The family says:

Phil: 'One of the most important things has been doing this together as a family – you are so much stronger as a unit. We used to turn it into a bit of a game – see who was losing most.

'It's changed our lives; we've broken our habits. I'd say most fat people know deep down what they should and shouldn't be eating but they can't put it into practice.

'Controlling your weight is 70% about what you eat and 30% exercise, you can't get away with changing one without the other.

'It's second nature to us now. We always start with a good breakfast – skip breakfast and you'll snack on something.

'We still have the odd takeaway but we have chicken tikka without the masala sauce, and plain rice instead of pilau rice. And when we cook curry at home we do it from scratch instead of using sauces from a jar.

'We've cut right back on the alcohol and I don't miss it – it just becomes a habit. I drink green tea with lemon during the day.

'And I'm never hungry – I eat enough of the right foods to fill me up, and I have healthy snacks. We haven't had any chips in eight months; I smell the grease and it makes me feel sick.

'One of the best things has been getting my life back – I've got so much more energy, I even do the washing up now. And I can buy my clothes in normal shops – I can get a T-shirt in M&S instead of forking out £30 for an outsize shirt that I might have had made for me.

'And Jan and I can get our arms around each other for a cuddle! We've got a king-sized bed and because we've lost almost 15 stone between us it's like we've lost a whole person out of our bed.'

Jan: 'The best thing has been the health improvements. When we had our last health checks Phil's liver was normal size, his diabetes is being controlled just by what he eats, and his and Kayleigh's cholesterol levels are down.

'We are just less worried every day about Phil's heart.

'It isn't difficult now, I feel I'm in control of my eating – I'm the gov'nor

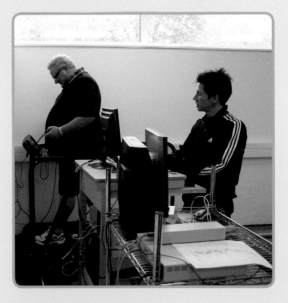

now! And when you know you're in control you can allow yourself the odd treat, the difference is you don't really want it any more. I look at a bag of crisps and remember that it'll take a long walk to use it up and I think I won't bother.

'In fact we don't even buy temptations now, we keep the house full of fruit and we keep ourselves busy.'

Kayleigh: 'I'm so much more confident now and I don't have to buy frumpy clothes, I can go into high street shops. And watching what my mum and dad have done has made it easier for me.'

The Huzzey family's top tips

- Get off your backside – there's always half an hour in the day when you can go for a walk, either during your lunch break or after dinner.

- Don't buy garments with elasticated waists – they stretch with you!

- Plan ahead and think before you eat.

- Don't drink alcohol during the week.

- Choose the healthier option off the menu.

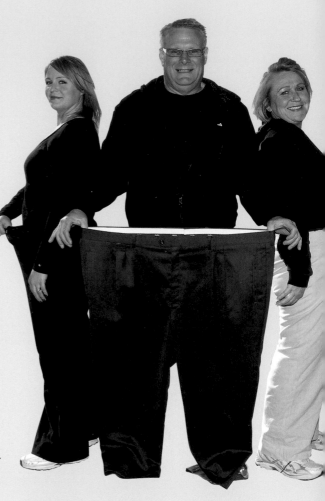

Party poopers

No one wants to give up having fun when they lose weight and it's often the thought of not being able to go to barbecues or have a few drinks that makes people give up a couple of weeks into their new healthy-eating plan.

But there are plenty of ways to still be the life and soul of the party without being the party porker.

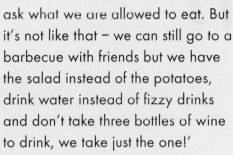

Booze busters

Remember:
1 bottle of wine = 550 calories = half a pint of cream
5 vodka cranberries = 19 shots of cream
6 pints of lager = 30 shots of cream

The golden rule is, never turn up to a party starving hungry, because the snacks are usually the worst foods there. A couple of handfuls of peanuts, crisps or tortilla chips with creamy dips and you've pigged out on fat, poor-quality carbs and salt, and you haven't even started eating yet!

- 25 g bag of peanuts = 160 calories
- 40 g bag of Extreme Chilli Doritos = 200 calories

And then the booze starts flowing ...

Apart from the fact that it's difficult to keep track of what you're drinking at a party if someone keeps on topping up your glass, it's even harder to remember that the glass of liquid is actually laden with calories.

Phil says: 'Some people are a bit funny when they invite us over and ask what we are allowed to eat. But it's not like that – we can still go to a barbecue with friends but we have the salad instead of the potatoes, drink water instead of fizzy drinks and don't take three bottles of wine to drink, we take just the one!'

Try imagining the booze as something else – you wouldn't down a half-pint carton of cream if someone offered it to you but that's roughly what you're doing when you enjoy a bottle of wine in an evening.

Try diluting white wine half-and-half with fizzy water into a spritzer. Some wines now are so strong – about 14% alcohol – that you could easily go over your recommended daily limit in one large glass.

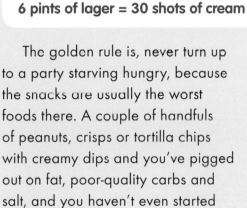

The Huzzey family

73

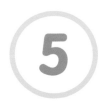

Eating healthily for life

So you've made the decision to turn your life around, you've cleared the junk food out of the freezer and the cupboards and you want to get started. But changing your eating habits can be hard unless you plan ahead.

Fat Families expert nutritionist Jessica Wilson worked with all the families on the TV series and says that although each family was different and had their own set of problems and temptations, the basic structure of planning and preparation of meals in advance works for everyone.

The absolute key to losing weight must lie in what you eat. Exercise is a very important part of a lifestyle plan and getting all the family up and exercising not only helps shift weight and makes everyone feel better but it's also a great way of spending time as a family. But realistically you cannot expect to eat excessively and then work it off in the gym – you would have to exercise intensively for hours and hours every day.

Whatever you are eating, the chances are you are eating too much of it, so portion control must be the first thing you look at. It's certainly the biggest problem in most families. Most people simply aren't aware of how much they should be eating – and usually they eat as much as the people they live with. They are guided by their eyes, not their stomachs.

'Mindless Eating'

An American called Brian Wansink discovered how easy it is to trick people into eating more food than they need – he called it 'Mindless Eating'. For instance:

• People who ate the same-sized portion from a small plate and a large plate thought they had eaten more from the small plate, and felt fuller.

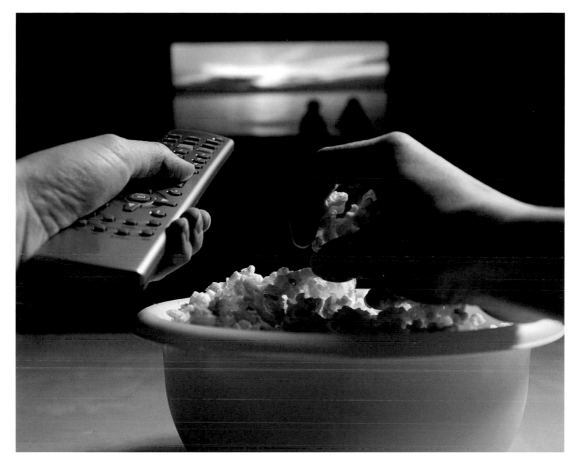

- People who ate soup from a bowl that was secretly being constantly topped up by a hidden pipe continued eating long after consuming a huge portion, simply because their eyes were telling them they hadn't eaten a bowlful.

- Cinema-goers ate more from an extra-large bucket of popcorn than a large bucket, despite there being more in the large bucket than anyone could finish.

The point is that we keep eating even when our bodies have actually had enough just because it doesn't occur to us to stop. That's why so many people eat massive amounts in front of the TV – it's because their mind isn't on what they are actually doing.

So get back in touch with your body and your appetite. Ask yourself whether you ever say, 'I must eat now because it's lunchtime/dinnertime', regardless of whether you feel hungry or not.

Planning and preparation

Think about what you are going to eat and shop for it. Plan meals and prepare snacks. How many times have you bought a chocolate snack or a bag of crisps from the canteen or vending machine at work because you felt peckish, when if you'd taken in some fruit you could have had a healthy bite instead?

Skipping breakfast in particular is a recipe for disaster – your body has been fasting all night and it needs an energy supply. Miss out breakfast and you'll hit the 11am biscuit crisis.

Breakfast doesn't have to be a time-consuming meal if you're on a tight schedule in the mornings; it can be quick and easy, but it's a must. But don't start the day with a sugary cereal – it'll raise your blood sugar quickly but it may crash down so you are tempted to pick at something sweet again. Breakfast should keep you going until lunchtime, with maybe an apple or a yoghurt in between.

PORTION SIZES

Are you piling your plate with food? Here are some visual guidelines for portions to help you make sure you're not eating to excess.

1 portion of:

- pasta/rice = a heaped handful
- potatoes = a computer mouse
- lean meat = a pack of cards
- fish = a cheque book
- cheese = a small matchbox

LEARN WHAT MAKES A MEAL UNHEALTHY

Are you one of those families who say they don't eat fattening food because 'We only have a bowl of pasta at night'? A huge bowl of pasta with a creamy rich sauce and probably grated cheese on top is not the same as a small bowl of wholemeal pasta with a tomato sauce and vegetables or a side salad. It isn't the pasta that's the problem, it's how much you eat and what you put on it.

Years ago, dieters were taught to count all the calories in everything they ate, but this method isn't a lifestyle that's easy to sustain. Of course you'll lose weight if you strictly count every calorie – you'll lose weight if you put any restriction on your eating – but what we're trying to do here is change your relationship with food so you can eat healthily but normally, without totting up what's on your plate.

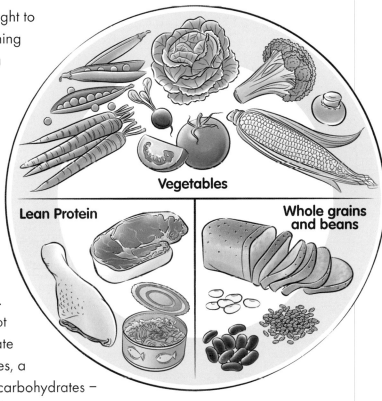

You should be in control, not the calculator. Ideally, your plate should consist of half vegetables, a quarter protein and a quarter carbohydrates – preferably whole grains, not white rice or pasta.

Don't be scared of fats but use minimal amounts of the good ones, such as olive oil or rapeseed oil, for frying and stay away from the baddies: saturated fats and the trans fats in processed foods (see pages 96–111 on food groups).

And if you're only using a small amount, there's nothing wrong with butter – it's not got additives, it's natural and it tastes better! If you're using margarines or spreads, make sure you buy those free from hydrogenated fats.

We have become obsessed with buying low-fat foods without checking on the label what else is in there. Low fat often means high sugar, a trick some of the 'diet' food producers know only too well. One household name 'diet food' producer makes a brand of low-fat oat digestive biscuits. They're

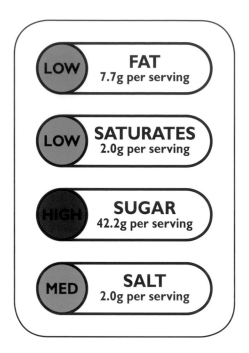

Nutrition information	
Typical values per 100g	
Energy	245kJ/58kcal
Protein	4.6g
Carbohydrate	7.2g
of which sugars	6.5g
Fat	1.2g
of which saturates	0.2g
Fibre	0.2g
Sodium	0.1g

(!) Allergy advice
May contain nut traces

low in fat all right, but actually have almost 4% more sugar than a McVitie's standard digestive.

Read the label!

Food labels are confusing! Here's a quick guide on how to read them. If the label has colours – known as the traffic light system – stay away from RED! It spells danger as it means the dish is high in that particular ingredient. Aim for foods with green or orange labels for FAT, SUGAR and SALT.

Take sugar as an example. (Figures are for every 100 g of food.)

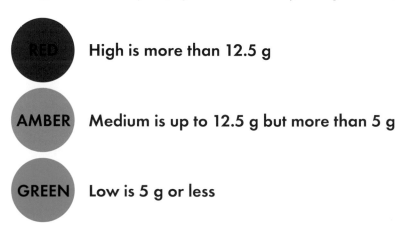

RED High is more than 12.5 g

AMBER Medium is up to 12.5 g but more than 5 g

GREEN Low is 5 g or less

Not every retailer uses the traffic light system so if the food just has a label with the nutritional information table on the side, the most important things to look for are the calories, sugar and fat contents per serving.

Always check the number of servings per packet so that you know what the intended portion size is (although do remember this is only the manufacturer's suggestion and it may be inappropriate). Portion control is one of the most important changes you can make in your new lifestyle.

And most of all, don't make excuses about your weight. Remember, most of your weight is within your control and just a small amount (some estimate around 20%) is down to things you can't control, such as genetics.

Children and eating

We all know that childhood obesity is on the increase and one of the most important reasons for losing weight and eating healthily yourself is that your children will be less likely to become obese and have the health problems that are associated with it.

Jessica Wilson's advice is not to put young children on diets – she wouldn't even put under-fives on skimmed milk. What they need is not a restriction on food but a new way of eating that will make them pleasantly full on good, nutritious food.

Children follow the eating habits they see at home. If plates are piled high, they assume that's how much they should eat. If the cupboards are stuffed with crisps and biscuits, that's what they will snack on.

There are two things you should cut out of their diets: sugary breakfast cereals and fizzy, sugary drinks.

Breakfast cereals aimed at children, such as the ones coated with chocolate, are just loaded with sugar – your child may leave the house in the morning having had their full daily allowance of sugar in one meal. Just swap to a lower-sugar variety and they can still have their hit of vitamins, minerals and milk.

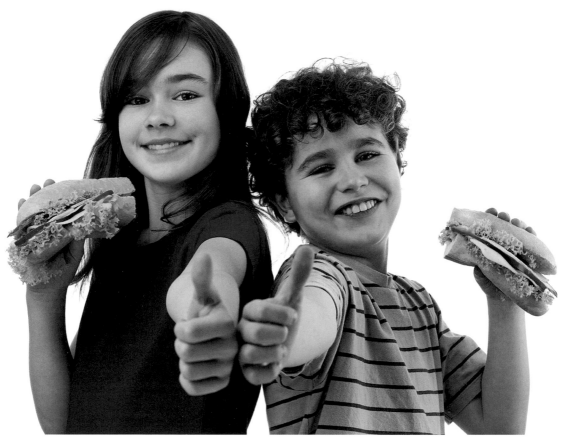

High-sugar fizzy drinks are just sugared water and have no nutritional value whatsoever. As well as contributing towards obesity, they are also creating serious health problems in children.

Studies have shown that heavy consumption of sweet fizzy drinks can deplete bone mass density, which in turn could lead to increased risk of osteoporosis and fractures. Part of the problem is that sweet fizzy drinks contain phosphoric acid, and because your body doesn't like being acidic, it will drain the calcium from your bones to neutralise this acid.

So unless it's a treat on meals out, get them used to drinking water (maybe with a twist of lemon), milk or diluted fruit juices.

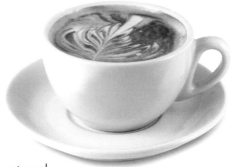

Keep a food diary

This is a good way to see exactly what you eat and
how much, but equally important when and why you eat.

- Do you fill up on milky coffee and a cake at 11am? Then perhaps
  you haven't had a proper filling breakfast.

- Do you have a sugar craving at three in the afternoon? Perhaps
  you've had a lunch high in carbohydrate and have 'crashed'.

- Do you fill yourself up with chocolate sitting in front of the TV
  at night? Maybe you're bored or unhappy, or just eating out of habit.

Don't forget to count in all the high-calorie coffees and sugary teas, or the
sugary drinks you have during the day. Lots of people ignore how much fat
and sugar they take in liquid form.

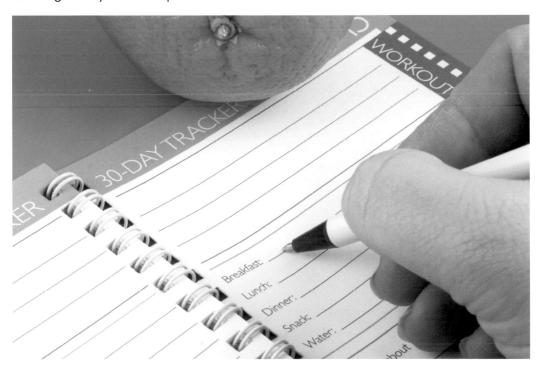

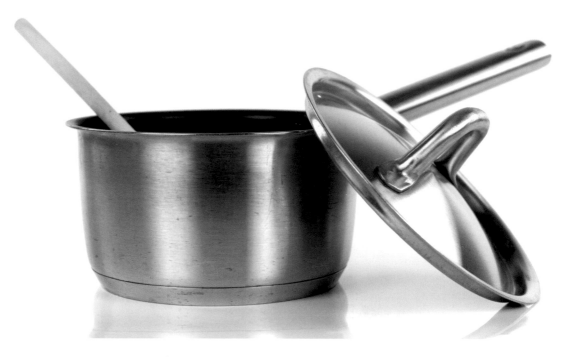

Do you cook?

Most of us feel short of time if we're juggling work and children, but you can be totally in control of what you eat if you prepare it yourself. No one expects you to come home every evening and rustle up a three-course meal, but it takes much less time than you imagine to prepare a tasty meal for two or for the whole family.

And if you have a freezer you can cook on weekends or days when you have more time and freeze portions to use during the week.

And turn eating into proper mealtimes around the table, not something you do standing over the kitchen counter or slouched in front of the TV.

If you eat around the table as a family, it will help you eat more slowly. Your children will see this and follow suit. Gulping down food doesn't allow your brain to catch up with the signals from your stomach that are telling you it's full.

Home cooking is a sure way of knowing what ingredients you are using – and how much. When you buy ready-made meals you have no control over what goes into them. A jar of tomato sauce may look healthy, but check the label for its sugar content.

A salad sandwich may sound healthy, but does it have a huge dollop of mayonnaise smeared inside?

And who decides what is an 'individual portion' of a ready meal? One size doesn't fit all, so is it for an athlete, a labourer, a young teenager or someone elderly? Don't be tempted into eating a meal that someone else has decided for you.

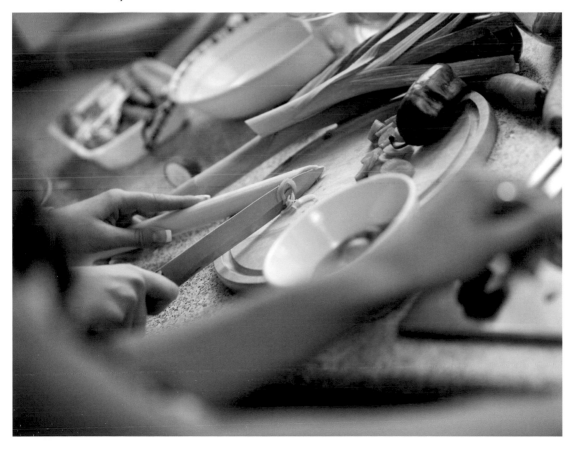

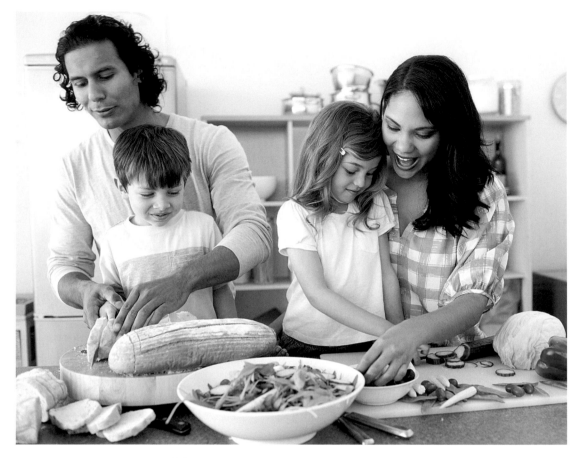

Treat yourself

Follow the 80/20 rule so that you can treat yourself:

> Eat healthy, small portions for 80% of the time and then, on a meal out or at a party, say, you can relax and have an extra glass of wine or a pudding.

You'll be surprised to find that once healthy eating becomes a way of life, fatty, sweet puddings or handfuls of crisps seem less tempting than they used to!

TIPS TO HELP YOU STICK TO THREE MEALS A DAY

1. Occupy your mind between meals. An occupied mind is a healthy mind, and will help to stop you grazing. Consider new hobbies and interests, or simply plan to do something that will keep you busy between meals.

2. Drink regular sips of water between meals. Feeling hunger often really means you are thirsty, so make sure you remain hydrated.

3. Be strong! Affirm in your mind that you are in control and are completely focused, driven and self-motivated to eat three meals a day.

4. If time allows, or on days you are home from work, do some exercise to fill time between meals. Simply go for a walk or pop to the gym.

5. Each day write a brief paragraph about how you successfully managed the day eating three meals. This will help to condition your mind for the long haul to stick to three meals.

6. Work out when you like to eat most. For instance, if you like to eat more at night, then have a small meal for breakfast and lunch and a hearty, healthy meal in the evening.

7. Eat slowly, remembering it takes around 20 minutes for the mind to be 'food satisfied'.

8. Forget making food the be-all and end-all in life!

The Joell-Ireland Family from Portsmouth

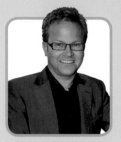

Steve visited the Joell-Irelands from Portsmouth.

'I'm on my way to meet a gargantuan couple whose greasy grub has got them sailing straight towards an early grave.

'Stephen and James are inseparable. They live together in their Portsmouth city apartment, they work together in a local call centre and more importantly they eat together. And when I say eat ... I mean eat!

'In their spare time they also run their own video-game review website, but this is even more disastrous for their waistlines.

'As a child, though, Stephen was a skinny tae kwon do champ until he hit his teens, when it all began to change.

'And until he met Stephen seven years ago, James was just 15 stone.

'So what went wrong to change these ordinary-sized lads into a juggernaut couple who are packing in a gut-popping 12,000 calories between them every day? That's the recommended calorie intake for four men and one woman!'

The stats (after 8 weeks)

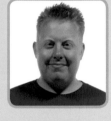

Stephen
Age: **26**
Height: **6' 4"**
Start weight: **26 st 11 lb**
Now weighs: **23 st 8 lb**

Total weight loss af: **3 st 3 lb**

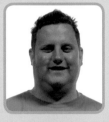

James
Age: **24**
Height: **6' 0"**
Start weight: **22 st 11 lb**
Now weighs: **19 st 10 lb**

Total weight loss: **3 st 1 lb**

Family's total weight loss: **6 st 5 lb**

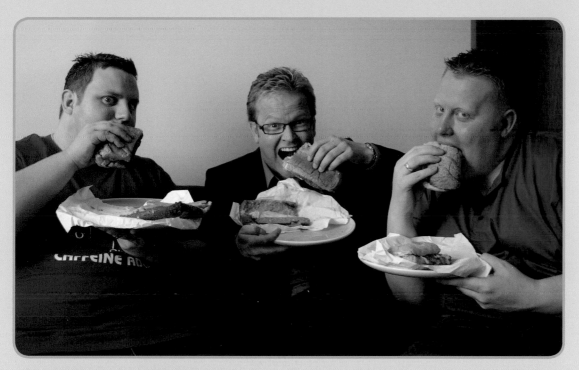

Main problem

Both men work long shifts at a call centre, where Stephen is a team manager, but they'd become too lazy to cook and ate nothing but convenience foods and takeaways. Living next door to a sandwich shop was the ultimate temptation. They would rather spend their time going out having fun than buying fresh food and cooking from scratch. James reviews computer games in his spare time, so often spends evenings hunched over a computer.

Neither did any exercise and when Steve Miller first made them swim in the sea, Stephen struggled to swim 15 yards. Because they live next to a sandwich shop they gorged on huge, foot-long filled rolls for breakfast, and James, in particular, drank gallons of high-energy drinks, which are packed with calories – 230 per can – and he's knocking back about five of these a day.

Stephen has a very sweet tooth and would snack all day on bags of sweets and in the evenings would eat tubs of ice cream.

Stephen had been skinny when he was young and neither have a history of weight problems in their families. They think they've become complacent since becoming a couple, especially since they got married in 2009.

Main motivation

Both were shocked by the medical, which showed that even at such an early age they were endangering their health. Stephen hadn't weighed himself for ten years, never looked in the mirror and bought his clothes from specialist online sites – his trousers were a 54-inch waist.

Steve Miller tore up one of their wedding photos and told them that if they carried on like this, one or other of them risked ending up alone. An early grave beckoned and it was a race to see who got there first. They had planned a future that might include adopting a baby one day and realised they were endangering all their dreams.

They also like singing and performing and wanted to look better to stand up in front of audiences.

Both of their families were very worried about their health and why they were putting on weight at such a rate.

Typical day's food: Stephen

Breakfast: Foot-long baguette, takeaway coffee with sugar, energy drink

11am: Sugary snacks, sweets

Lunch: 2 sandwiches or burger, crisps, chocolates, fizzy drink

3pm: Coffee with sugar, energy drinks, sweets

Dinner: 2-inch-thick pizza, chicken wings, garlic bread and potato wedges

Late-night supper: Microwave burger

Medical tests

We ran tests on both men and found that, despite their young age:

James: Had raised levels of uric acid in his blood, which can lead to the painful joint condition, gout. He already had signs of fatty liver disease and was warned that his

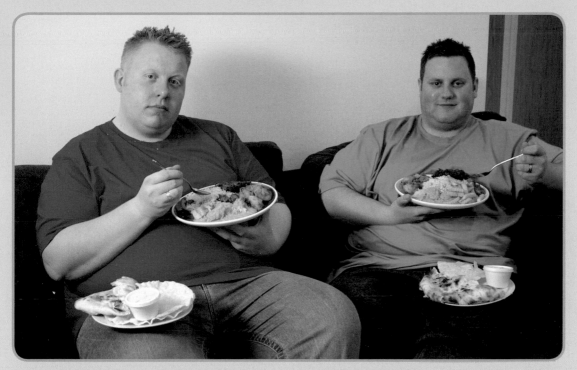

poor health would probably lead to heart problems. His body fat percentage was 48% – that means he was carrying 70 kg of fat.

Stephen: Was warned he also had high uric acid levels in his blood and was heading for heart problems. His body fat percentage was 56% – that means he was carrying 95 kg of fat.

Lifestyle changes

Stephen and James are intelligent young men with lots of plans for the future, but were stuck in a gluttonous rut where they were bad influences on each other. James used to be much lighter and tried to encourage Stephen to lose weight, but they ended up growing bigger together and using their long hours as an excuse. But they had plenty of time to sit in front of the computer in the evening, when James reviews computer games.

Steve Miller said, 'They're young 20-something blokes but they're pretty much confined to their sofa like old men. I'm surprised they haven't got bed sores.'

They needed to:

1. Get some time management so they could forward plan and not use lack of time as an excuse

2. Learn to cook fresh meals from scratch

3. Cut back on portion sizes

4. Cut back on sweets (Stephen) and energy drinks (James)

5. Start doing some exercise

6. Drink more water instead of assuming they were hungry when really they were thirsty

Exercise regime

Neither Stephen nor James did any exercise at all, despite living near a wonderful coastline, where they could go walking or swimming.

Personal trainer Bernie Saupe said, 'They were both young so had plenty of time to turn things around but they had a totally sedentary lifestyle – even their spare time was spent sitting playing computer games.

'But their competitive habits played to their advantage – they liked the idea of spurring each other on and fortunately they are losing weight at a roughly equal rate.

'The first priority was weight loss, so we started with cardiovascular activity to get their heart rate up, so they would use the cross trainer, do some rowing and jog a bit. They started off lightly but by the third week the pace was increasing and when the weight started to shift they needed to do some weight training and press-ups to start toning up the muscles. Strength training gives some shape when the fat drops off and helps tone flabby arms. They used weights, went hill-climbing and did some boxing-pad work. Some of these exercises keep the brain tuned up too.

'Variety is important – there's no point just using the treadmill for hours on end. And as they love computer games they could make use of games on the Wii Fit or use the Tour De France simulation programmes in the gym.'

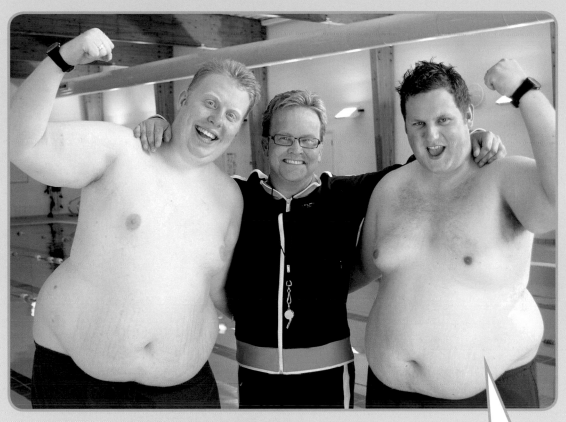

James: 'I thought I was bionic until I had to come face to face with what I had done to my body. It was a terrible shock to think we might lose each other.'

They go to the gym two or three times a week and use an exercise bike at home every day. They also have an exercise ball that they sit on to play computer games so they have to use their abdominal muscles to stay balanced. For the first time they now also go swimming and take long walks.

James: 'On the first week, my body was adjusting to doing exercise and my leg muscles were tight so I could manage only about ten minutes a day. But it's amazing how soon you get into it and just make it part of your life. I can even be on the exercise bike now when I'm reviewing a computer game and sometimes, if it's a driving game or something, it actually makes me go faster!'

Stephen: 'This whole regime has boosted my confidence. I would never have gone to a public swimming pool before – now I just

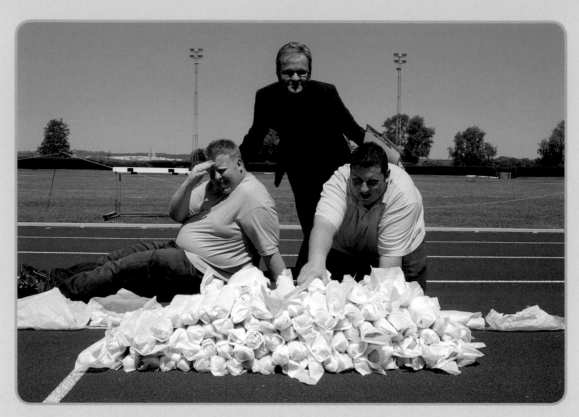

think I don't care what people see, I'm on my way and my confidence is sky-high. Steve set us a swimming challenge of 500 metres in our local pool and he was worried we wouldn't make it – but it was a breeze! I think he should have set us something harder!'

Healthy eating

Jessica Wilson was appalled at the breakfasts the Joell-Irelands ate – a foot-long baguette with sugary coffees or energy drinks was about 1,500 calories – before the day had even begun! And James was drinking at least five energy drinks a day while sitting on his bottom!

And although the couple worried that fresh food was expensive, in fact it has turned out to be cheaper. They are saving money and can spend it on clothes and going out instead of wasting it on huge fatty curries that will one day kill them. Portion plates were a huge incentive so they could see just how much they should be eating at each meal – and it came as a gigantic shock.

James didn't seem to have a clue how to prepare food except for things like beans on toast, so Jessica gave him some cookery lessons.

Stephen took to cooking with great enthusiasm and now will cook up a batch of vegetable soup, which he freezes for use later in the week.

Jessica showed how they could add vegetables to everything they ate to increase their fibre and vitamin intake – as well as adding herbs and spices to give sauces, soups and even salads a bit of extra zing.

Cutting back on the huge proportion of fat in their diet was a priority and when Steve laid out 100 metres of foot-long fatty baguettes – the equivalent of three each per week for a year – Stephen and James were almost speechless at seeing what they actually ate.

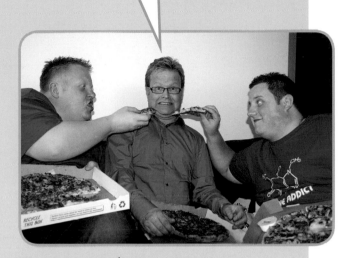

going to control my eating – I was conscious of what the hospital trolley was bringing round and I managed, despite everything going on, to still lose weight that week. So what started as a downer ended up as something I was proud of!'

Progress highs and lows

Stephen: 'About week four or five I suffered one of my cluster headaches (excruciatingly painful attacks of head pain) and I had to be hospitalised for three days – it completely knocked me out. While I was in my hospital bed I was determined that I was still

James: 'I didn't cope very well when Stephen was taken into hospital – I rely on him a lot so I fell back a bit that week and didn't lose my target three pounds. In fact, I slipped into bad habits and I remember having leftover curry on toast for breakfast one morning!

'But I got back on track and the next week I lost seven pounds! So mine went from low to high as well.'

Fatty fizzers

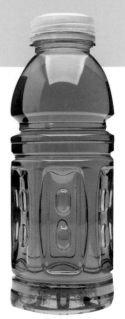

In Britain, we knock back nearly half a billion litres of energy drinks a year and, like James, most of us don't actually need that extra boost of energy because we're doing nothing to burn it off. It's like buying expensive gym equipment and lying in bed all day, except the gym equipment harms only your bank balance, not your heart!

- Two cans of energy drink contain the same amount of sugar as one and a half strawberry gateaux.

- To burn off two cans of sugar-laden fizz you would need to do lunge stretches for an hour and a half.

- Many energy drinks contain high levels of caffeine, which can stimulate your heart and cause sleeplessness and irritability.

The family says:

Stephen: 'James and I are a team and we needed each other to do this. We have so many plans for the future; we want to travel and maybe eventually adopt a baby, so we know that this is our chance to change.

'And now so many more things are opening up to me just through losing weight. I always wanted to play those arcade games where you sit in a car and drive a track but before I was too big – the feeling when I was first able to do it was incredible. I can start to see the rewards for what I'm doing and I've set myself new targets – I want to go skydiving! I haven't had an energy drink in eight weeks.

'Each week I see the scales and it gives James and me an even closer bond to be doing this together. James's mum always worried so much about our weight so it's wonderful to be able to show her that we are doing this for real.

'And at work I don't think I realised how much people judge you for being fat until I started to lose weight.'

James: 'I can't believe how much more energy we have now – I was always tired before but I've just been for a 12-mile trek along the

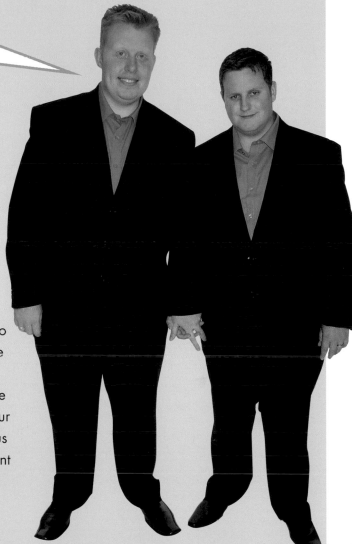

Stephen: 'Convenience foods comes at a price and we've found out what it is. We were living in denial.'

coast of the Isle of Wight. This has turned our lives around. We don't even want to eat the stuff we used to live on before – our taste buds have changed and we want things that have more flavour that actually taste of food. When Steve mulched up our favourite pizza with oil and made us taste it – that was a real turning point for me. It was disgusting.'

James and Stephen's top tips

- Enjoy what you're doing and think about it as something positive.

- Remind yourselves of all the things you will be able to do better when you're slimmer and fitter – we've booked a holiday.

- Set each other targets.

- Go swimming – you're not too big and it's good for overall fitness. Don't worry what anyone else thinks.

- Swap fizzy energy drinks for fizzy water with a slice of lemon.

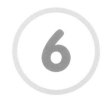

What are you eating?

The nutrients that make up the food we eat are divided into three main categories: proteins, fats and carbohydrates. They all have different jobs in the body and we need some of each group in a balanced diet to help us perform those jobs. So cutting out all fats, for example, is depriving the body of essential nutrients.

What does each of these groups do and where can we find them?

Proteins

Proteins are the building blocks of our body – they are the second most common components in the body (after water) and are used to grow and repair our body as we use it – that's why it's a good idea to eat protein after exercising to help restore muscle.

Enzymes, which are essential for many chemical reactions in the body, are proteins, as are many hormones, like adrenaline and insulin.

Most of the protein we eat in our Western diet comes from animal sources – meat, fish, eggs and dairy products – but we can also find it in plants. All proteins are made up of smaller units called amino acids – there are about 20 in all but 8 of those are what are called essential amino acids, that is we need them for our bodies to function properly. The body can't manufacture these, so we must take them in as food and as we digest the protein it breaks down into amino acids.

Animal protein sources contain these eight essential amino acids but plant protein sources may only contain some of them.

That's why animal protein is known as 'complete' protein. But vegetarians can build all the amino acids into their diet by eating different combinations of plant proteins, e.g. pulses and grains together, such as baked beans (pulse) on toast (grain). On their own, pulses are short of the amino acid

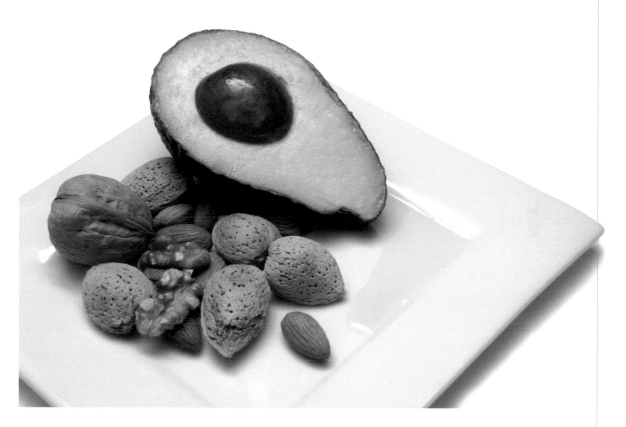

methionine and grains have lower levels of lysine and tryptophan, but together they provide all eight essential amino acids.

Sources of plant proteins include soya, nuts, seeds, pulses, avocados, grain foods and Quorn.

Low-carbohydrate diets, such as the original Atkins Diet, relied on a high protein intake and virtually no carbohydrates. It can kick-start fast weight loss but eating large quantities of protein over a long period may put a strain on the kidneys and can make the body's internal environment more acidic. That acidity has to be neutralised so the body uses its own calcium, taking it from the bones. So, yet again, our bodies are telling us that a balanced diet keeps it functioning best.

It's rare in this country to eat too little protein; you actually only need small portions to provide enough in the diet, though it varies according to age and body size.

Fats

Poor old fat has become the bogeyman of healthy eating. Cut out fat, we are told, as it will kill you.

But the problem is that there are all sorts of different fats — some of which we very much need and others we certainly don't.

We need fats because:

> **FACT**
> The average man should consume no more than 30 g of saturated fat a day, the average woman no more than 20 g. But if you are losing weight, you should aim to keep your saturated fat levels as low as possible.

• A lot of our body is actually made up of fats. Our brain and nervous system, for instance, is made up of about 60% fat.

• Vitamins A, D, E and K are soluble only in fat.

• They keep our skin supple and hydrated.

Fats come in three basic types: saturated, polyunsaturated and monounsaturated, depending on the way the molecules which make them up are bonded.

Saturated fats are the ones that get all the bad press. They're found in meat and dairy products and are used to make buttery products like cakes and biscuits. They are usually solid at room temperature (butter, lard, etc.).

Polyunsaturated and monounsaturated fats are found mainly in nuts, seeds and some plants. They stay liquid at room temperature and many of them aren't suitable for heating to very high temperatures as that changes the structure of the oil and makes them potentially damaging to your health.

Olive oil is a great all-purpose oil as it can be used for cooking and in salad dressings.

But let's look at the real goodies and baddies of fats.

The baddies: trans fats

The real baddies of the fat family are hydrogenated oils and fats, which start out as unsaturated fats but have hydrogen forced into their chemical bonds. This is to give them a longer shelf life so they can be used in making processed foods that don't need refrigerating. In the process of hydrogenation, a fat called trans fat may be created and these have been linked to high cholesterol and cardiovascular disease.

Trans fats don't have to be included on food labels, so it's best to avoid foods with hydrogenated oils, which do have to be put on the label.

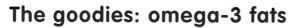

Many major supermarkets are banning trans fats from their own-brand foods, but they're often used in the fast-food industry for frying.

The goodies: omega-3 fats

The good fats that we need more of in our diet are omega-3 fatty acids, which are found mainly in oily fish such as salmon, mackerel and sardines. These oils help fight inflammation in the body, maintain a healthy nervous system and may help to protect against coronary heart disease. But because most people in this country don't eat one portion of oily fish a week – the suggested amount – most of us have a low intake of this fatty acid.

And vegetarians obviously eat even less. There are good sources of omega-3 in walnuts, flax seeds, soy beans and rapeseed oils, but the body has to convert these oils into the most useful form and that conversion process is not very effective. So vegetarians would have to eat a large quantity of these nuts and seeds for the body to manufacture enough omega-3s. There are some flax-seed-based supplements available to help this, but again they aren't very effective.

Carbohydrates

Carbohydrates come in two sorts: simple and complex.

Simple carbohydrates are forms of sugar in single units, while complex carbohydrates, or starches, are more complex joined molecules of sugar. In food terms, the best form of complex carbs are foods in a more natural, whole-grain state, such as whole-grain bread, rice and porridge oats. Simple carbs, on the other hand, are more processed and refined, such as white bread and flour, breakfast cereals and cakes.

The main purpose of carbohydrates is to provide energy for the body in a very efficient form. We need this energy for everything, from breathing to running, and we need it 24 hours a day.

When we eat carbohydrates, they are broken down into a sugar product called glucose, which travels in the bloodstream to wherever it's needed. If it's not needed there and then, it's stored in the liver and muscles as glycogen. But when the liver and muscles are full up, it gets turned into fat.

The reason complex carbohydrates are much better for us than simple carbohydrates is that they release their energy more slowly and evenly.

A release of glucose from carbs triggers the pancreas to release a hormone called insulin, which then transports the glucose into cells such as muscle cells. If we eat too many simple carbs that release glucose quickly, the pancreas has to work harder to step up the production of insulin to deal with the glucose. The more simple carbs you eat throughout the day, the more the insulin is released, and this can disrupt the balance of the blood sugars. Eventually, your body may stop responding properly to the insulin and become resistant to it, which is the first step on the path towards type 2 diabetes.

The excess glucose in your system will eventually have to be turned into fat –

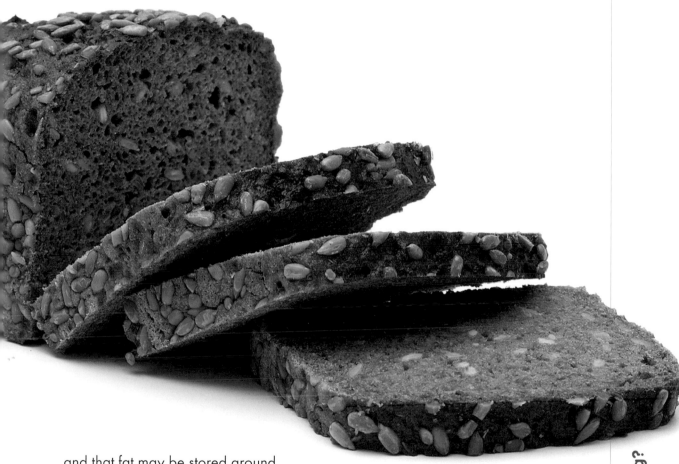

and that fat may be stored around
your middle – the 'muffin-top' band of abdominal fat.

By changing your diet to include whole-grain complex carbs instead of refined ones, you allow the insulin to work more efficiently and your body won't experience the energy peaks and troughs.

In Western diets, much of the fat in our diet has been replaced with a high intake of carbohydrates in the belief that this is healthier. But some nutritionists claim that the sort of carbohydrates we're eating – white bread, pasta, sugary breakfast cereals, croissants, muffins, biscuits – is contributing towards the rise in type 2 diabetes.

Sugar

Sugar is one of the most refined types of carbohydrate so deserves a section of its own.

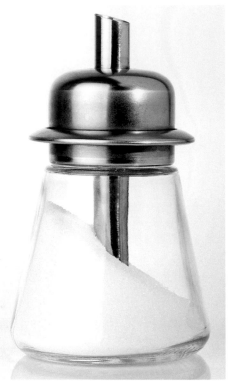

The problem with sugar is that we don't know how much we are eating because it's hidden in so many foods. You might avoid it in your tea and coffee but find it's lurking in your Indian chicken tikka masala takeaway ...

We get plenty of sugar from natural sources in our food, so we don't need to add more to our diets. There are three types of sugar in food:

- **Intrinsic sugars** are those contained naturally within the cell structure of all our fruit and vegetables. You don't need to worry about these because they come as part of a package of vitamins, minerals and fibre that is good for our health.

- **Milk sugars** (lactase) are sugars that occur naturally in milk and milk products, and you don't need to worry too much about these because they're part of a healthy protein and calcium package.

- **Non-milk extrinsic sugars (NME)**, which are the sugars added to food to sweeten them, preserve their shelf life or bulk them up. These are the ones that do most of the damage, lurking in fizzy drinks, cakes, breakfast cereals and even some savoury foods like peanut butter and baked beans (though not all brands).

Food manufacturers love sugar because it's cheap – and we love the taste so it makes many foods taste even better.

And beware of the misleading food labelling – sugar comes under many different names. Manufacturers know that we prefer to think of honey as natural and healthy – and it may have some some health benefits – but it's still just sugar when it gets inside your body!

Fibre

Fibre is that part of carbohydrate foods our bodies can't digest and there are two types, soluble and insoluble.

Both types can be found in fruit, vegetables, pulses and grains. The insoluble fibre, as its name suggests, passes through the digestive system pretty much untouched whereas soluble fibre is converted to a sort of gel inside the intestines.

Fibre is part of a healthy diet because it helps to speed up the movement of food through the intestines and prevents constipation. Some sorts of fibre, such as that in porridge oats, can also lower your LDL (bad) cholesterol level.

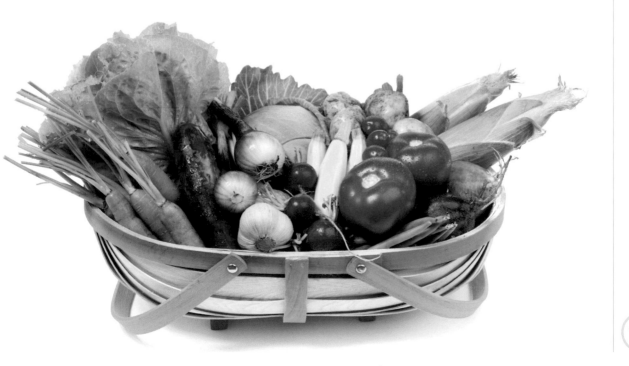

Good sources of fibre are beans, peas, lentils, whole-grain foods and most fruit and vegetables.

A diet rich in processed foods probably lacks fibre, so when you change to a healthier diet you may find that your bowel health improves.

Vitamins

Walk into any chemist and you'll see shelves full of vitamin supplements promising all sorts of health benefits. And the chances are that when you've had a cold or felt a bit run down, you've taken some extra vitamin C or a multi-vitamin.

But the truth is that although supplements can certainly play a part in boosting a poor diet, you should be able to get all the vitamins and minerals you need from your own food – with the bonus of the other nutrients that come from the food.

Some vitamins, such as vitamins B and C, are water-soluble so anything extra you take that your body doesn't need you will just pee away! But this also means that you can't store them, so you need to eat food rich in these vitamins regularly.

Others are fat-soluble – A, D, E and K – which means your body stores them in fat cells and the liver. Rarely, taking too many of these vitamins can create a build-up in your system, causing health problems. Again, sticking to a balanced diet should mean you don't take in too much of any one vitamin.

If you vary your food as much as possible, include fresh fruit and vegetables at every meal (stick some tomato and cucumber in that cheese sandwich!) and eat some animal protein or a vegetarian source of protein such as tofu, Quorn or nuts every day, you should be hitting your vitamin and mineral targets.

So let's have a look at why you need each vitamin in your body.

Vitamin	Needed for	Good sources	Deficiency can cause
A	Healthy immune system, normal bone and teeth growth and maintaining good vision	**There are two sorts:** (1) Retinol comes direct from animal products such as liver, egg yolks, dairy products and mackerel (2) Carotenoids come mainly from red and yellow fruit and vegetables (carrots, pumpkin, tomatoes, etc.), and are converted into vitamin A in the body	Dry, dull skin and hair, poor wound healing, problems with mucous membranes causing ulcers, sinus problems, acne and poor vision, especially at night
B^1 (Thiamine)	Releasing energy from food, plus healthy working of heart, cardiovascular system, nervous system, muscles and mucous membranes	Whole grains, chickpeas, brewer's yeast, kidney beans, liver, peas and peanuts	Fatigue, depression, poor mental function, cramps, nausea and poor digestion
B^2 (Riboflavin)	Releasing energy from food, healthy brain, nervous system, hair, skin, nails and keeping mucous membranes in good order	Dairy products, yeast extracts, eggs, wheat germ, green leafy vegetables, bananas, beef liver and tuna	Red, cracked mouth and tongue, fatigue, depression, scaly skin – especially on the face, anaemia and poor digestion with constipation or diarrhoea

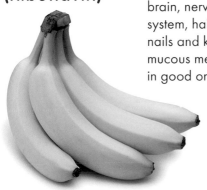

What are you eating?

Vitamin	Needed for	Good sources	Deficiency can cause
B^5 (Pantothenic acid)	Forming a coenzyme involved in metabolism of fats, proteins and carbohydrates	Nuts, egg yolks, green leafy vegetables, bananas, lentils, whole grains and most meat	Dizziness, nausea, constipation, excessive fatigue and muscular weakness
B^6 (Pyridoxine)	Healthy nervous and muscle systems, skin, hair and red-blood-cell formation, metabolism of energy from protein and carbohydrates	Chicken, sunflower seeds, oily fish, wheat germ, oatmeal, eggs, dairy produce and soya	Skin problems, mental confusion, irritability, anaemia and depression
B^{12} (Cobalamin)	Makes red blood cells, maintains healthy nervous system, helps process folic acid, releases energy from foods	Meat, algae such as seaweed and blue-green spirulina, salmon, shellfish, milk, cheese and eggs	Anaemia, fatigue and lack of mood control
Folic acid (B complex)	Involved in the creation of DNA, so vital for a developing foetus, building red blood cells and immune cells, metabolises protein and carbohydrate energy	Green leafy vegetables, asparagus, avocados, Brussels sprouts, wheat germ, carrots, apricots and citrus fruit	Anaemia, mood disorders, fatigue, gastrointestinal disorders, furring of arteries, and can contribute towards neural tube defects in a developing foetus
Biotin	Releasing energy from fats and proteins, healthy skin, hair and nails	Egg yolks, lentils, mushrooms, nuts, brown rice, brewer's yeast, liver, cheese and oatmeal	Dermatitis, eczema, anaemia, muscle pain, lethargy and hair loss

Vitamin	Needed for	Good sources	Deficiency can cause
C (Ascorbic acid)	Tissue repair, building immune system, cardiovascular health, nervous system, absorption of iron and calcium, healthy gums and teeth, healthy sperm production	Citrus fruit, all berries, tomatoes, kiwi, green peppers, broccoli, spinach, watercress and Brussel sprouts	Frequent infections, poor wound healing, bleeding gums, anaemia, nosebleeds, bruising, weak muscles and skin problems
D	Helps to absorb calcium and phosphorus to build strong bones, maintains healthy nervous and immune systems. Has been linked to reduced risk of some cancers, including bowel and breast	The best source of vitamin D is sunlight, which is absorbed through the body and used to make vitamin D internally. Also found in bony fish such as mackerel and sardines, cod-liver oil, eggs and dairy products	Weakened teeth and bones, bone and muscle ache. Severe deficiency can cause rickets (soft, curved bones) in children
E	Protects against cell damage, improves the immune system, helps normal growth and development, healthy skin	Avocados, almonds, brazil nuts, sunflower seeds, wheat germ, soya beans, broccoli and olive oil	Lethargy, anaemia and dizziness
K	Normal blood clotting and kidney function	Asparagus, broccoli, Brussels sprouts, Cheddar cheese, seaweed, spinach and liver	Easy bleeding and bruising

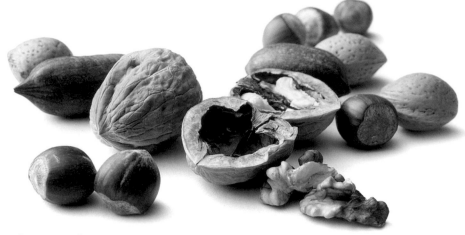

Minerals

Minerals are chemical elements that are essential for the body to function properly. They help to build bones, enable red blood cells to carry oxygen around the body, digest food, regulate blood pressure, blood sugar, hormones and fluid levels, and help to maintain the nervous system. The most likely inadequate intake in modern diets are iron, calcium, selenium and zinc.

We need some in larger amounts, others only in trace amounts.

Mineral	Needed for	Good sources	Deficiency can cause
Calcium	Builds strong bones and teeth, helps blood to clot and muscles to contract, regulates the nervous system and blood pressure, and the secretion of hormones. Note that vitamin D is needed to absorb calcium	Nuts, dairy products, soya beans, broccoli, eggs, dried fruit, watercress and bony fish such as sardines	Osteoporosis, high blood pressure, muscle cramps, and has been linked to an increased risk of colon cancer
Chromium	Works with insulin to help regulate blood glucose levels and cholesterol levels. Cardiovascular health. Helps maintain healthy skin, bones, muscles and hair	Meat, egg yolk, cheese, whole grains, nuts, seeds, beetroot, asparagus and brewer's yeast	Blood-sugar fluctuations, irritability, fatigue, sweating and dizziness

Mineral	Needed for	Good sources	Deficiency can cause
Iodine	Production of thyroxine, the hormone that regulates the thyroid gland that helps to control weight, energy, metabolism and healthy hair, skin, teeth and nails	Kelp, seafood, seaweed, blue-green algae, sea salt, milk, eggs and meat	Obesity, constipation, slower mental processes, cold feet and hands. Can also cause goitre, a swelling in the thyroid gland
Iron	Making red blood cells, helping to carry oxygen and also essential for the immune system	Red meat, seafood, eggs, raisins, nuts, seeds, lentils, dried fruit, soya beans, parsley, broccoli and green leafy vegetables	Very common, especially among women, leading to anaemia. Tiredness, paleness, cracks at corners of the mouth, coldness, muscle weakness, palpitations and brittle, ridged nails
Magnesium	Works in a delicate balance with calcium in building bones, metabolising essential fatty acids, thyroid function, regulating nerve and muscle function, cardiovascular health, helps sleep and relaxation	Green leafy vegetables, mushrooms, wheat germ, avocados, nuts, seeds, legumes, whole grains, onions and garlic	Muscle tics, tremors, hyperactivity, sleeplessness, palpitations and anxiety

Mineral	Needed for	Good sources	Deficiency can cause
Manganese	Control of blood-sugar levels, production of thyroid and female hormones, making haemoglobin, healthy nervous system, efficient use of vitamins, bone repair	Brown rice, pulses, nuts, eggs, avocados, pineapple, banana, coffee, quinoa and tea	Rare, but could cause low blood sugar, poor bones and cartilage
Phosphorus	Builds healthy teeth and bones, metabolises energy from food, repairs cell and tissue damage and activates the B vitamins	Milk, meat, poultry, fish, legumes and eggs	Muscle weakness and loss of appetite
Potassium	Regulates the flow of fluids in and out of the body, helps to control blood pressure, heart and kidney function, maintains healthy nervous system	Green leafy vegetables, sesame seeds, soya flour, lentils, fish, bananas, mushrooms, almonds, melon, apricots and chicken	Can cause thirst, fatigue and muscle weakness, palpitations and dry skin
Selenium	Boosting immune system, supporting liver and cardiovascular system, working with vitamin E as an antioxidant. Helps to promote healthy skin, hair and nails	Seafood, liver, kidneys, brazil nuts, broccoli, garlic, tomatoes, lentils, chickpeas, seeds and mushrooms	Frequent infection, fatigue, poor wound healing, increased risk of infertility and heart problems

Mineral	Needed for	Good sources	Deficiency can cause
Sodium (salt) 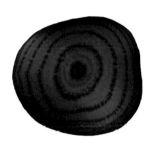	To work with potassium and chloride to regulate movement of body fluids, transmit nerve impulses, relax muscles, regulate blood pressure and the body's acid/alkali balance	Root vegetables, dairy products, bread and processed foods	Unlikely – we generally eat too much salt! But levels can be reduced by diarrhoea or sweating, causing cramps
Zinc	Wound healing, healthy skin, boosting immune system, production of insulin, digestive functions and sperm production	Seafood, meat, liver, turkey, whole grains, nuts, seeds, legumes, buckwheat, brown rice, tofu and ginger	Skin problems, loss of appetite, ulcers, bacterial infections, poor wound healing and possible low sperm count

People at risk

Certain groups of people are more at risk of vitamin and mineral deficiencies than others, so should up their intake of the right foods:

- **Vegans and strict vegetarians ...**

   ... may be deficient in vitamin B^{12}, which comes mainly from animal sources. Try soya milks fortified with B^{12}, or cereals with this added vitamin.

   Vegans and vegetarians may also be low in iron. Iron from non-animal sources isn't absorbed as efficiently by the body, so always eat or drink something rich in vitamin C when eating iron-rich foods, such as a glass of fresh orange juice, as it helps the body absorb it. (Women who have monthly periods can also have low iron levels.)

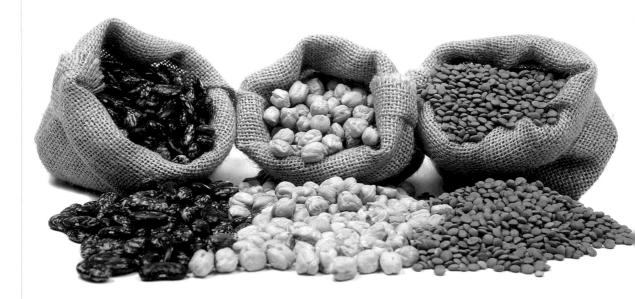

Zinc is another mineral that can be at low levels in vegans, so add a tablespoon of pumpkin seeds to smoothies or salads, or just snack on a handful. Don't worry that they're quite high in calories, all that oil is the good sort!

Vegetarians often replace meat and fish with cheese, which can make their diets high in saturated fat. Try other protein sources such as beans, pulses and soya.

• People who rarely go out in sunlight ...

... can be deficient in vitamin D, because radiation from the sun stimulates the production of vitamin D in the body. This includes groups who cover up in public for cultural reasons and people who never go in sunlight without a strong sunscreen. The further north you live, the less likely you are to get sufficient exposure to sunshine.

Although the risk of cancer from overexposure to the sun is very real, it's important to let unprotected skin get some sunlight every day, if possible. You don't have to bask in the sun – around 20 minutes is plenty – and fair-skinned people need less exposure than the darker-skinned. And you can't absorb the rays needed through glass, so sitting by a window doesn't count!

- **Teenagers who go on 'exclusion' diets ...**

  ... tend to cut out whole food groups such as dairy products. The teenage years are vital for laying down stores of calcium in the bones, so adolescents need to eat a diet rich in calcium. If you don't eat dairy, make sure you eat other calcium-rich foods such as canned salmon and sardines (with bones), cabbagge, almonds, broccoli and fortified soya products.

- **Smokers ...**

  ... may have lower levels of vitamins C and B^{12} – yet another reason to give up!

- **Alcoholics and heavy drinkers ...**

  ... may have low levels of vitamins B^1, B^2, B^6, B^{12}, C and folic acid.

- **People who take antacids or who drinks lots of tea ...**

  ... may not absorb iron as efficiently. The antacid medicine and tannins in tea hamper the absorption of iron. Try drinking herbal teas instead, which do not contain tannins, or drink it away from mealtimes.

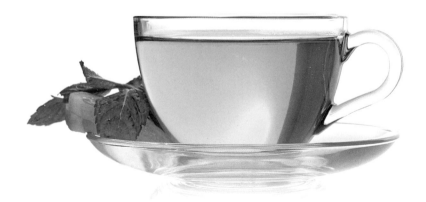

These are the building blocks of your diet and each food group plays an important part in keeping you fit and healthy. Also a healthy diet is as varied as possible so vary what you eat for breakfast, lunch and dinner. Ring the changes for a greater range of nutrients – it will stop you getting bored and succumbing to temptation!

The Haddrell family from Luton

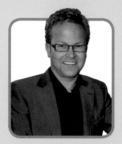

Steve visited the Haddrells from Luton in Bedfordshire.

'The hefty Haddrells didn't just snack between meals – they would meal between meals. They spent their lives cramming their faces full of fatty takeaways, processed foods and super-sized sweet treats.

'If this lardy lot had been able to stick to three meals a day they wouldn't have needed my help – but they couldn't.

'The Haddrells chomped their way through 20,000 calories a day!'

The stats (after one year)

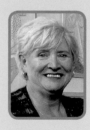

Mum: **Eileen**
Age: **49**
Height: **5' 6"**
Start weight: **21 st 11 lb**
Now weighs: **17 st 9 lb**

Total weight loss: **4 st 2 lb**

Auntie: **Linda**
Age: **58**
Height: **5' 9"**
Start weight: **18 st**
Now weighs **14 st 11 lb**

Total weight loss: **3 st 3 lb**

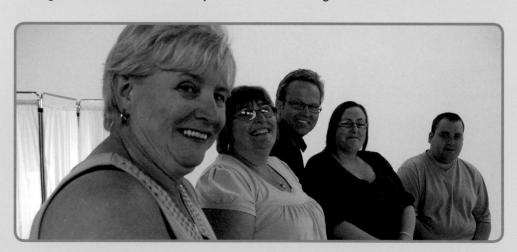

Daughter: **Sarah**
Age: **23**
Height: **5' 6"**
Start weight: **21 st**
Now weighs: **17 st 3 lb**

Total weight loss: **3 st 11 lb**

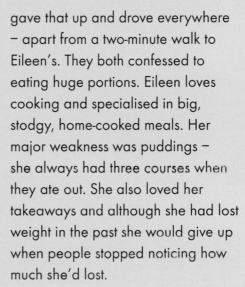

Son-in-law: **Matthew**
Age: **24**
Height: **5' 8"**
Start weight: **17 st 8 lb**
Now weighs: **12 st 10 lb**

Total weight loss: **4 st 12 lb**

Total family weight loss: **15 st 10 lb**

Main problem

Newly-weds nursery nurse Sarah and aviation security officer Matthew had been overweight since childhood and as both work full-time they lived off convenience foods, takeaways or Mum Eileen's big roast dinners.

They both admitted to being lazy and in the past had given up diets very easily. They joined a gym but gave that up and drove everywhere – apart from a two-minute walk to Eileen's. They both confessed to eating huge portions. Eileen loves cooking and specialised in big, stodgy, home-cooked meals. Her major weakness was puddings – she always had three courses when they ate out. She also loved her takeaways and although she had lost weight in the past she would give up when people stopped noticing how much she'd lost.

Matthew and Eileen also admitted to being secret eaters – Matthew will sometimes have a burger on the way home before dinner.

Auntie Linda also loves cooking for the family but hated waste and would polish off leftovers before bed. She lives alone but still shops as though she has a family at home.

Main motivation

Matthew and Sarah want to try for a baby but knew they needed to lose weight and get healthy before starting a family of their

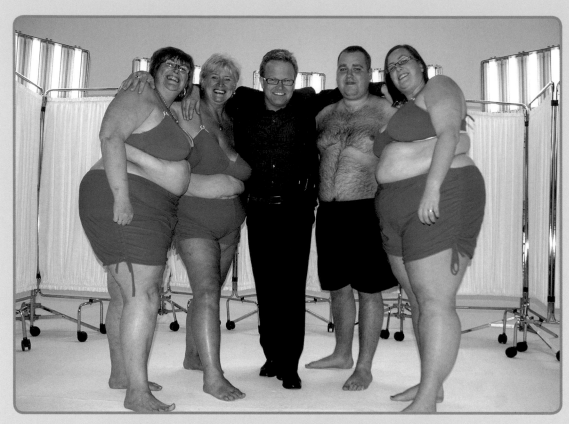

own. They knew that they wanted to break the fat cycle so they don't bring up their future children to be overweight.

Being young, they were also fed up of not being able to buy and wear trendy clothes – they felt they looked old before their time.

Linda looks after her husband (who is in a care home) and needed to be fitter and healthier to cope.

Typical day's food: Sarah

Breakfast:	Buttery toast
Mid-morning snack:	Crisps, 3 chocolate bars
Lunch:	Pastie
Dinner:	Large portion of chicken Kiev and chips with garlic bread, or fast food or Chinese

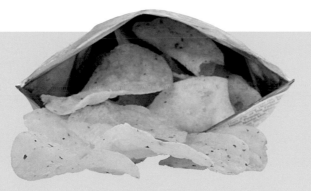

Medical tests

We ran tests on the Haddrells and discovered that:

Matthew: 42% of Matthew's body was pure fat (in men, it should be between 10 and 20%). He had high blood pressure, high cholesterol and central obesity, i.e. fat around his middle. That meant that at just 24 he'd already got three major risk factors for a heart attack.

Sarah: Sarah's body-fat ratio was even worse at 58% (in women, it should be no higher than 33%). If she had become pregnant, then she ran the risk of high blood pressure and pregnancy diabetes, which could have put both her and the baby's health at risk.

Linda: Linda's body was 46% fat and needed to drastically reduce. She was already on lots of medication for weight-related illnesses and her eating habits were just making her problems worse.

Eileen: She was carrying a whopping 59% body fat and was already showing signs of fatty liver disease. She risked developing more serious liver problems if she didn't change her life. Those sweet treats had to go!

Lifestyle changes

The Haddrells are a very close, loving family but Steve was worried about their determination levels. He said, 'What concerns me most is that it's like you guys have befriended fat. When I talked to you about fat there was lots of laughter.'

But they came out fighting, determined to prove Steve wrong.
They needed to:

1. Get off their bottoms and move. Matthew and Sarah in particular are far too young to be so inactive

2. Ditch the puddings

3. Bin the convenience foods and takeaways

4. No more secret snacking in between meals

Exercise regime

By their own admission, the family was very lazy when it came to exercise and didn't really like the idea of going to a gym and exercising in front of other people.

Personal trainer Dave Coard didn't want them closed off in a little room; he preferred to get them outdoors, so they compromised and turned the back garden into a private gym!

Dave says, 'The first night I met them we did just a half-hour assessment, a bit of shadow boxing, slow jogging and a few exercises that raised their arms above their heads. We kept talking all the time because that way people breathe naturally, they don't hold their breath or tense up.

'Matthew really got into exercise – he liked the more masculine stuff, doing circuits, press-ups, and loved the boxing. He was really focused and I knew once the weight started to come off that all the exercise would really boost his self-confidence. He's done so well, I think he could start training for a marathon.

'I know Eileen hit a bit of a barrier but that's quite common, that's why I try to change the exercise routine every six weeks because it gets stale. Weight drops off very quickly and then it might stick for a couple of weeks and people get disheartened, but they have to remember how much they have lost and how much their fitness has improved and get back on board.

'In the garden we did circuit training as if we were in a gym: hand weights, skipping, bench presses, running on the spot, step-ups. Sarah underestimated what she could achieve – she needed to be pushed that little bit to do a press-up because she didn't believe she could.

'And when they wanted to stop for a breather I'd encourage them to keep moving. Even when you stop, you can still walk around, swinging your arms.

'It's supposed to be fun so doing it in a group or as a family makes it sociable.'

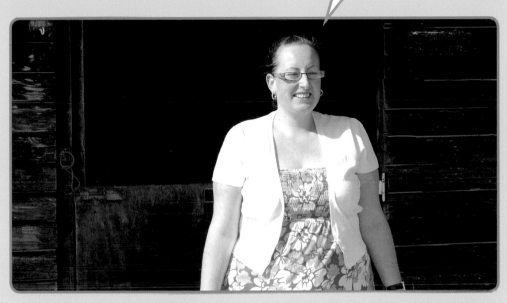

Sarah: 'I don't want to stay fat, especially if I want to be a mum. I don't want to be a fat mum.'

Matthew has been totally converted. 'I preferred more manly stuff to the water Aquafit the girls like, so I've done a lot of running and weights work to tone up my body as the fat dropped off.'

Healthy eating

Jessica Wilson said, 'One of the problems here was a sweet tooth, especially for Eileen, so we had to wean her off the sugary stuff. You need to change your taste buds and that doesn't happen overnight, you can't go cold turkey. You have to start getting used to the naturally sweet taste of real fruit instead of sugared foods and cut out fizzy drinks.

'Eileen never really needed a pudding at the end of a meal – it was just habit.

'And Matthew had to stop sneaking in the extra meals on his way home – once he adjusted to a healthier diet he didn't actually have those sudden hunger crashes which are to do with poor blood-sugar control.

'Because they are a close family and like cooking and eating together, they could start giving up takeaways and taste home-cooked food with lots of flavours.

The Haddrell family

'They all knew what they were doing was making them fat, they just needed to be pushed out of their lazy habits.'

Progress highs and lows

Eileen hit a crisis in week seven when she stopped losing weight. She swore she had been following the food plan to the letter but admitted that she hadn't been exercising. Most people will hit a wall at some time but at least Eileen recognised it and called for help. Being diagnosed with a fatty liver was a real wake-up call and she wasn't giving up this time.

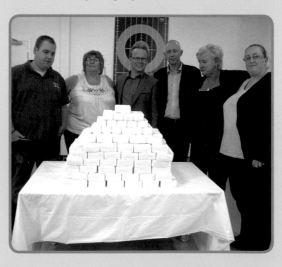

The family says:

Linda: 'Steve has stopped me getting old. I have a new lease of life, I'll be 60 in March and I feel like I'm 40 again. My husband has Parkinson's and is in a care home, and he calls me his slim, brand-new wife!

'When you live alone it's harder to motivate yourself but the family has been a tremendous support. My clothes size has gone from 28 to 20 – but my new problem is that I love shopping so much now that my kids have threatened to take my credit card away!

'I was on 18 tablets a day for my health problems, now I take 3. My blood pressure is under control, I don't take tablets for diabetes any more and my cholesterol is down.

'I've stopped buying enough food for a family and now buy for myself – then there's no waste to eat up.

'To be honest, I haven't found this hard – I have had to exercise against my normal regime, which was dictated by hip problems, but I took on board what the trainer suggested

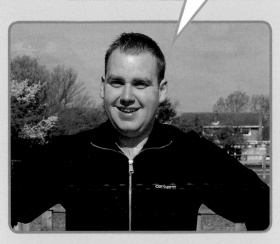

Matthew: 'I'm feeling more confident, more sexy, more of an achiever. I can set my sights and do anything.'

and I do the Aquafit every week and walk the dog every day.

'This hasn't been a diet, it's been a life-changing programme for me.'

Eileen: 'The most important thing for me has been the family support – I've tried losing weight before and just cheated – now if I'm having a bad week there's someone to support me – we do it together.

'We go to aquaerobics every week and I do Wii Fit, whereas I did nothing before. I drove everywhere, searched out the parking space nearest to the shop, used lifts. There's nothing I miss about my old life. I think I've always been confident outwardly but this has lifted my internal self-esteem.'

Sarah: 'My confidence is boosted and I feel more comfortable in who I am. Matthew and I go for walks together and we can talk and have time on our own instead of sitting in front of the TV.

'And it's lovely to be able to go into a normal shop to buy clothes, not an outsize store. I think having all the family doing it together was the key thing for me.'

Matthew: 'It's changed my life. I get treated with more respect at work and am included in more things – I even get flirted with now! The hardest thing was giving up all the burgers and snacks – it was such a habit it felt like giving up smoking, something my body craved. But I don't even think about them now. I eat three meals a day and have a few healthy snacks.

'I think I'm about my ideal weight now so I need to monitor it. It makes it a bit harder for Sarah because I can now eat some stuff that she can't allow herself but she's determined to keep going.'

The Haddrell family

Sweet temptations

For people like Eileen sweets and chocolates can prove too tempting to give up. Steve taught her to imagine a piece of chocolate was covered in her least favourite foods: in Eileen's case cottage cheese and jellied eels! Every time she was about to pop a piece of chocolate in her mouth she pictured it covered in lumpy white cheese or slimy eel – and it made her want to gag!

- Just ten squares of chocolate = a quarter of your recommended daily saturated-fat intake.

- If you're going to treat yourself to some chocolate, it is better to eat small pieces of better-quality dark chocolate – it has a higher proportion of cocoa solids and sugar. It's more expensive and has a stronger flavour but also has potential health benefits!

- Avoid filled chocolates – most of that filling is just flavoured sugar.

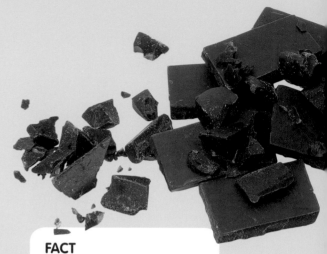

FACT
In Britain we chomp our way through £3.5 billion of chocolate every year.

The Haddrell family's top tips

- Make exercise part of your social life – join a class together and treat it like a night out. We girls go to Aquafit once a week.

- Keep to a routine so you're not tempted to give it a miss – that's simply the day you exercise, so get on with it.

- Don't make excuses – there aren't any.

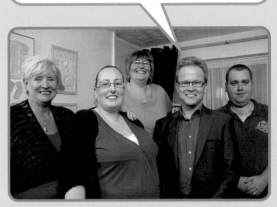

Steve: 'I've been so impressed with your focus and motivation. I feel I've made four friends.'

- Shop only for what you are going to eat – if you live alone, then you don't need much. And throw away leftovers straight away.

- Push yourself just a bit further than you think you can go when walking, running or swimming – don't stay in your comfort zone.

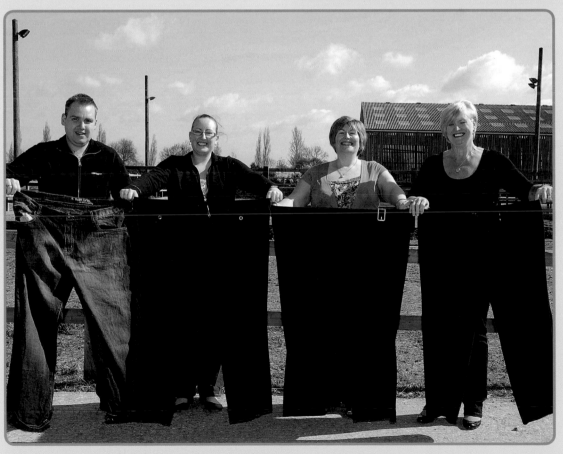

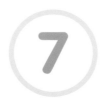

Lowering your cholesterol

One of the many problems associated with obesity is that people who are very overweight tend to have high cholesterol levels. As described on page 31, high levels of LDL cholesterol can be damaging to the heart and cardiovascular system so it's important to try to bring down these levels while boosting the levels of HDL, which can protect against heart attacks.

What should I eat?

Although we need some cholesterol, the liver produces all we need, so you can affect (to some degree) your cholesterol by what you eat. You should cut out high saturated fats, and in particular the artificial trans and hydrogenised fats. You can also help your cholesterol by eating foods that have been shown to actually lower LDL. Latest research shows interesting results from the foods below, so it might be worth adding them to your new eating plan.

Porridge

A steaming bowl of porridge in the morning doesn't just give you a good start to the day – it could be performing a mopping-up operation on excess cholesterol.

Porridge oats are a form of soluble fibre that has been proven effective at lowering cholesterol levels. Porridge contains a fibre called beta glucan, which attaches to bile acids in the

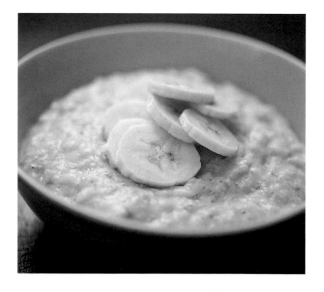

intestine, causing them to be excreted – the body then uses up some of the cholesterol travelling around the bloodstream to make more bile acids.

Having 60–80 g of porridge oats a day can lower cholesterol by 10%. Ideally make it with water or, if that's too spartan for you, use skimmed milk to keep the fat content down. And add some fresh berries or half a banana.

Oily fish

Oily fish such as mackerel, salmon and herring are all rich in omega-3 oil, which is thought to offer protection against heart disease by raising HDL and lowering the harmful fats.

Vegetarians can find omega-3 oils in flax seeds and walnuts, but the body needs to perform an extra conversion process to gain the benefit from the oil, which can be slow.

If you want to take an omega-3 supplement, make sure it contains sterols and stanols (see below).

Sterols and stanols

These are plant-based substances similar to human cholesterol and, because doses of around 2 g a day have been shown to reduce LDL by around 10%, they are being used in various foods such as certain soft cheeses, margarines and yoghurts. They do, of course, occur naturally in foods like avocado or rice bran but you would have to eat these in huge quantities to get a protective effect.

Lots of brands now advertise the fact they include plant sterols and stanols, but make sure you use them as part of a low-fat eating plan.

Soya

There are many health claims for soya – and some critics of it – but it is generally accepted as having cholesterol-lowering properties. Research suggests that 25 g of soya protein a day could have an LDL-lowering effect.

Good sources include tofu, tempeh (bean paste), soya yoghurts and soya milk (preferably unsweetened). Soy sauce has high salt levels, which may affect people with high blood pressure. Use it sparingly and look for reduced-salt types.

Use unsweetened 'lite' soya milk to make your morning porridge for a double-whammy strike at that fatty enemy!

Anything else worth a try?

There's no conclusive evidence that the following foods reduce cholesterol, although many nutritionists believe they do, but they are certainly worth a try as they may have other positive health benefits.

Turmeric root (curcumin)

This member of the ginger family, used widely in Asian cooking to give that lovely, rich yellow colour and pungent aroma and taste, is thought to inhibit cholesterol absorption in the intestines.

Use pure turmeric root if possible, stored in the fridge, or the dried powder, stored in an air-tight container, rather than a general curry-powder mix, as levels of curcumin in these can be very low. Mix in with yoghurt and use on raw vegetables or in cooking curries. Please note, this is not an excuse for ordering high-fat Indian takeaways!

Curcumin is delicious mixed with oil and ginger to cook salmon or chicken – always use black pepper when you cook with turmeric (as it helps the body absorb it better). It has long been used as an anti-inflammatory in Indian medicine and is currently being investigated as a treatment for Alzheimer's.

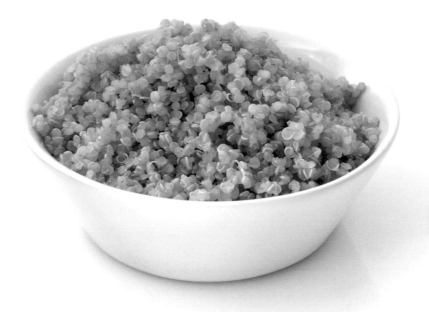

Quinoa

This much under-used type of superfood is packed with protein and nutrients, and helps fight high cholesterol. Used instead of rice, it soaks up flavourings and is very filling without being fattening.

CoQ10 AND STATINS

Coenzyme Q10 is a vital chemical present in every cell in the body, but levels do go down with age and it can be seriously depleted in those taking statins to lower cholesterol. Some studies show Q10 can reduce LDL if taken as a supplement, as it prevents the oxidisation that causes the fat to harden. Check with your doctor before taking supplements if you are on medication or have any health conditions.

Don't panic if your cholesterol reading is high – it isn't a sign of an imminent heart attack, but it is a sign that your body needs some attention. You may need to look at improving your lifestyle in other ways – get more exercise, drink less alcohol and quit smoking (if you do so) – rather than just changing what you eat.

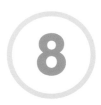

Meal planning

In this chapter you'll find some great recipes to make healthy, delicious meals for you and your family. But first, here are some simple guidelines from *Fat Families'* nutritionist Jessica Wilson to help keep you on the right path.

EIGHT GOLDEN RULES FOR HEALTHY EATING

1. Eat three square meals a day and make sure you eat breakfast every day.

2. Never skip meals. If you do, you'll either snack too much or overeat later.

3. Manage those portions! Follow our plate guide on page 77.

4. Add lots of vegetables to your meals to fill you up. You can eat as many vegetables (except potatoes) as you like. Swap traditional spuds for sweet potatoes.

5. Switch from white bread and pasta to 100% wholemeal bread or wholewheat pasta. This will fill you up and keep you fuller for longer. An added advantage is that 'brown' foods will help to keep you regular!

6. Switch from full-fat to semi-skimmed milk.

7. Don't eat the skin or fat on meat.

8. Don't deep-fry food.

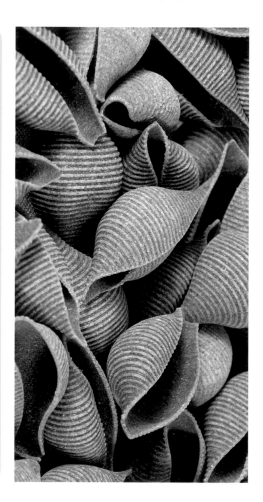

SIX FOODS TO AVOID

1. Fast food and takeaway food
2. White bread, including French baguettes
3. Fizzy drinks – some great alternatives to follow!
4. Cakes and biscuits, including pastries
5. Crisps and any salted nuts
6. Sweets and chocolate (unless specified below)

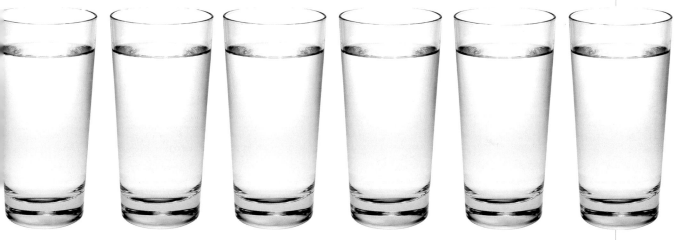

Body-friendly drinks

You might think you're hungry when actually your body is just thirsty. You should be drinking six to eight large glasses (about 1.2 litres) of fluid a day. Water is the best hydrator, but you can also count in:

- Herbal teas – experiment with different flavours until you find one you like
- One small glass of pure fruit juice per day – or dilute it with water and have two glasses
- In a perfect world, you should swap fizzy 'pop' drinks for fizzy water. For flavour, add fresh lemon, lime or orange slices. It's great for the skin too!

FIVE TIPS FOR EATING OUT

Eating healthily doesn't mean you have to stop going to restaurants. Here are some tips for finding food on the menus that won't pile on the pounds:

1. Choose chicken or fish dishes.

2. Avoid anything fried or with a cream sauce.

3. Ask the waiter to give you salad dressing or sauce on the side, then you can add just a little and save lots of calories.

4. Ask the waiter not to add butter to your dishes.

5. Choose a non-creamy soup to start; it fills you up and stops you from eating the extras.

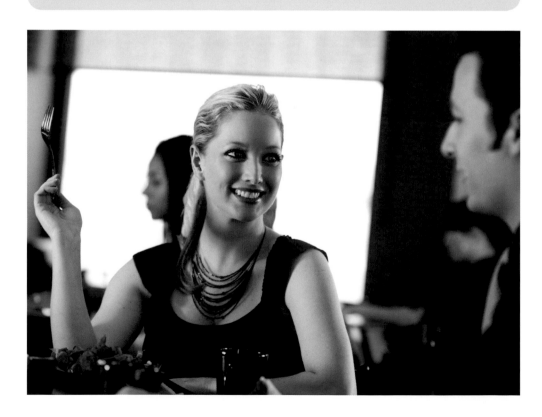

Taking control

To make it easier to get started on your eating for a new life, we're giving you the same meal plans that food expert Jessica Wilson gives the families on the show, so that – until you get into the swing of planning and preparing your own meals – you can follow the suggestions she makes here. The meals, devised by Jessica, are all healthy, filling and simple enough to make for even the most reluctant cook! The menu plans are for three meals a day.

Day 1 menu plan

Breakfast
Cereal (see page 134).

Lunch
Chicken sandwich: two slices of wholemeal bread with one cooked chicken breast (skin removed) and one sliced tomato or any other vegetable (spinach, watercress, cucumber). You can add mustard or a teaspoon of light mayonnaise. One apple.

Dinner
Coconut chicken curry (see recipe on page 142) and an orange.

Day 2 menu plan

Breakfast
Porridge (see page 134).

Lunch
Bowl of soup (any kind without cream). One piece of wholemeal bread or roll. Two small slices of low-fat cheese. One apple.

Dinner
Spaghetti bolognese (see recipe on page 143). One scoop of low-fat ice cream.

Day 3 menu plan

Breakfast

Egg on toast (see page 134).

Lunch

Baked potato (small) with baked beans and salad. Bowl of strawberries.

Dinner

Fish pie (see recipe on page 145). One orange.

Day 4 menu plan

Breakfast

Bacon, tomatoes and mushrooms (see page 135).

Lunch

Tuna, cucumber and low-fat soft-cheese sandwich on wholemeal bread. One apple.

Dinner

Two lamb chops (grilled). Three small new potatoes. Large helping of steamed broccoli and carrots. One scoop of low-fat ice cream.

Day 5 menu plan

Breakfast

Sugar-free muesli (see page 134).

Lunch

Small baked potato with a small handful of grated low-fat cheese and a large salad.

Dinner

Grilled chicken breast with lime and soy sauce. Stir-fry vegetables and 60 g of whole-grain brown rice.

Day 6 menu plan

Breakfast

Mushrooms on toast (see page 135).

Lunch

Greek salad, including mixed salad leaves, tomatoes, cucumber and a small helping (40 g) of feta cheese. Add a salad dressing (see page 138).

Dinner

Chilli con carne with rice (see page 144). One orange.

Day 7 menu plan

Breakfast
Fruit salad and yoghurt
(see page 135).

Lunch
Small portion (60 g) of
wholewheat pasta with tuna and
sweetcorn. One piece of fruit.

Dinner
Grilled chicken with mash
(see page 141).

Snacks

If you are hungry you can have up to
two snacks per day. Choose from:

- 1 piece of fruit with 1 tsp of
  pumpkin seeds
- 2 oatcakes/2 rice crackers/
  some raw carrots with 2 tbsp of
  hummus
- 1 small pot fruit yoghurt
- small handful unsalted nuts and
  dried fruit

FOUR TIPS FOR LOW-FAT COOKING

The way you prepare your food can have a big impact on how
healthy it is. Here are some tips for reducing fat in your cooking:

1. Steam your vegetables if you can, otherwise boil lightly.

2. Never deep-fry anything!

3. Bake and grill if you can. Try not to fry but if you do … steam-
   fry. It sounds weird, but use a teapoon of olive oil in a non-stick
   pan to start and then add a splash of water or stock (chicken or
   vegetable). The food cooks just as well in the water and oil; you
   save calories and it tastes great.

4. Otherwise, use an olive oil spray in a non-stick pan, as this really
   cuts down the amount used.

Meal planning

133

Breakfasts

All these breakfast portions are per person. You can vary them as much as you like. Why not save the bacon for a weekend reward – but only if you've not cheated the rest of the week!

Cereal

Two Weetabix or two Shredded Wheat with semi-skimmed milk. You can add chopped unsalted nuts or fresh fruit (half a banana is great).

Egg on toast

Two eggs per person. Boiled, scrambled or poached is great. Two slices of wholemeal toast (with a tiny scraping of butter or spread). A glass of pure fruit juice (150 ml juice maximum with 150 ml water) and a small tin of baked beans (go for the reduced-sugar, low-salt version).

MEASUREMENT GUIDE:
tsp = teaspoon
tbsp = tablespoon

Sugar-free muesli

A medium bowl (50 g) and always go for the no-added-sugar versions. You can add more chopped fruit like strawberries for sweetness. Semi-skimmed milk, obviously, and, if you like it, three tablespoons of plain natural yoghurt.

Porridge

Use 60 g of plain porridge oats with 300 ml of semi-skimmed milk. Add chopped nuts and fruit if you like. Instant oats are fine, but definitely not the flavoured varieties, as they're loaded with sugar and hidden calories.

Peanut butter on toast

Two slices of wholemeal toast and sugar-free peanut butter. Don't go mad with it, though – just spread it on thinly! Plus an apple.

Mushrooms on toast

Fry 200 g of mushrooms, sliced, in a non-stick pan with olive oil spray or half a teaspoon of olive oil. Stir in two tablespoons of low-fat cream cheese, add a grinding of black pepper and serve on two slices of wholemeal toast (with a tiny scraping of butter or spread).

Bagel with smoked salmon

Something for the weekend! Toast a brown bagel and lightly spread with low-fat cream cheese and 30 g of smoked salmon. Add a squeeze of lemon juice and black pepper.

Bacon, tomatoes and mushrooms

Reward yourself – but only if you've been good all week – with a healthy cooked breakfast. Grill two rashers of unsmoked bacon and remove the fat before you serve up, with grilled tomatoes and mushrooms cooked in a little olive oil. If you like ketchup, switch to the low-sugar, low-salt version and don't go mad with it!

Fruit smoothie

Grab your blender. Bung in two handfuls of berries (the packs from the supermarket freezers are great and not too expensive). Add 150 ml of semi-skimmed milk, 2 tablespoons of plain, natural yoghurt, 50 ml of apple or orange juice and half a small banana. Blend.

Fruit salad and yoghurt

Cut up a mixture of your favourite fruits, such as strawberries, blueberries, apple and pineapple. Add a small pot of low-fat plain yoghurt. And, if you want, a teaspoon of honey.

A note on breakfast cereals

Weetabix, Weetabix Oaties and Shredded Wheat are all okay, but take care to stay away from sweet breakfast cereals, as they're loaded with calories! (Check the box to see how much sugar a cereal contains – you might be surprised!)

Lunch ideas

Select your lunch from the ideas on the next few pages, and add a piece of fruit. Choose from: apple, orange, pear, plums (have two), a small banana or a bowl of berries.

Sandwich or small baked potato fillings

Have two slices of wholemeal bread, one wholemeal pitta or a small baked potato with one of these fillings:

Chicken: one small cooked chicken breast (skin removed) and one sliced tomato or any other vegetable (spinach, watercress or cucumber).

Smoked mackerel: one small smoked mackerel or trout fillet with a smear of low-fat cream cheese and watercress.

Salmon: 120 g (small tin) of canned salmon, mackerel, sardines or tuna in brine, with tomato, cucumber and cress. Add one teaspoon of light mayonnaise and lots of lemon juice and black pepper for flavour.

Egg: egg 'mayonnaise' (made with two hard-boiled eggs, a teaspoon of light mayonnaise, a tablespoon of cottage cheese, chopped spring onion and salt and pepper).

Hummus: 150 g of hummus with lettuce and grated carrot.

Soups

Soups are perfect to make in batches and freeze in portions. And they're not just for the winter, either: you can have hearty, warming soups in the winter or light, chilled ones in the summer.

Have one portion of soup from the recipes below (if you're eating out, make sure you choose a soup without cream). Serve with a large salad (mixed leaves, cucumber, tomatoes, peppers) with two teaspoons of salad dressing.

Vegetable soup

Serves 4

1 tbsp olive oil

2 onions, peeled and chopped

2 sticks celery, finely chopped

1 leek, sliced

2 tsp dried herbs (thyme, rosemary, basil)

1 tsp ground coriander

1 tsp smoked paprika (optional)

850 ml vegetable or chicken stock

450 g mixed root vegetables (carrot, butternut squash, parsnip), peeled and chopped into bite-size chunks

2 x 400 g cans mixed pulses (or beans of your choice, such as kidney, chickpea, borlotti, butter or flageolet)

Fresh flat leaf parsley

½ tsp salt and freshly ground black pepper

1. Heat the oil in a large pan. Sauté the onion, celery and leek until soft. Stir in the dried herbs, coriander and paprika (if using). Add the stock and the root vegetables.

2. Cover and bring to the boil, then reduce the heat and let the soup simmer for 20 minutes.

3. Stir in the mixed pulses, then cover and simmer for 5–10 minutes until the vegetables and beans are tender.

4. Add the parsley and check before seasoning. Try not to add more salt!

Minestrone soup

Serves 4–6

1 tbsp olive oil

1 onion, peeled and chopped

2 garlic cloves, peeled and finely chopped

2 medium carrots, peeled and sliced

1 stick celery, sliced

400 g can chopped tomatoes

1 tbsp tomato purée

2 litres chicken or vegetable stock

200 g wholewheat pasta shapes

1 bay leaf

1 tsp dried thyme

300 g frozen peas

Salt and freshly ground black pepper

Freshly grated Parmesan (1–2 tsp per person)

Fresh basil (optional)

1. Heat the oil in a large pan. Sauté the onion and garlic gently for 5 minutes. Add the carrots and celery and cook for a further 5 minutes. Add the tomatoes, tomato purée, stock, pasta, bay leaf and thyme. Bring to the boil, lower the heat and simmer for 15 minutes.

2. Add the peas, bring back to a simmer and cook for a further 5 minutes. Remove the bay leaf, season to taste and add the Parmesan and chopped basil to serve.

Salads

Salads don't have to be boring! You can put all sorts of things in a salad to make it taste good. Add a great dressing like the one below and you'll want to eat salads all the time!

Salad dressing

1–2 tsp per serving

5 tbsp olive oil

2 tbsp balsamic or wine vinegar

1 tsp French mustard

1 garlic clove, peeled and crushed

Salt and pepper

Mix all the ingredients together in a jar and shake before serving.

Delicious

The recipes that follow are quick and easy to make and can be made as soon as you come in from work. Finish off with a piece of fruit for a healthy, filling dinner.

REMEMBER YOUR PORTION CONTROL!

The following recipes are for four people. If you're cooking for two, save half and refrigerate for the next day.

Prawn or chicken stir-fry

Serves 4

1 tsp olive oil

1 large garlic clove, peeled and crushed

200 g large prawns, peeled and deveined (fresh or frozen) or 200 g skinless, boneless chicken breast, cubed

50–75 ml vegetable or chicken stock

dinners

1 red onion, peeled and sliced

1 red chilli, deseeded and finely chopped (optional)

Thumb-size piece of fresh ginger, peeled and finely sliced

100 g beansprouts

75 g green beans

75 g sugar snap peas

2 carrots, peeled and finely chopped

1 red pepper, deseeded and chopped

1 courgette, sliced

2 tbsp soy sauce

Juice of 1 lime

25 g cashews or plain peanuts, chopped (optional)

Fresh coriander (optional)

240 g cooked brown/white rice (60 g per person)

1. Heat the oil in a wok or large non-stick frying pan. Add the garlic and stir-fry for a couple of minutes.

2. If using prawns, stir-fry until pink all over (approx 1–2 minutes). If using chicken, cook until the meat is golden brown all over (approx. 5 minutes).

3. Add a splash of stock and the onion, chilli (if using) and ginger. Stir-fry for 2 minutes.

4. Add the rest of the vegetables and more stock if necessary. Stir-fry for a further 3 minutes.

5. Stir in the soy sauce and lime juice and stir-fry for a further minute. Sprinkle on the nuts and coriander (if using) and serve immediately with the rice.

Stir-fries are a great way to eat lots of tasty veg, plus they're really easy to cook in just a few minutes.

Cheesy pasta bake

Serves 4

250 g wholewheat pasta shapes (e.g. rigatoni or penne)

1 tbsp olive oil

1 red onion, peeled and finely chopped

200 g mushrooms, sliced or chopped

75 g sugar snap peas, halved lengthways

125 g spinach leaves

150 g low-fat soft cheese

175 g cottage cheese

Salt and freshly ground black pepper

4 tomatoes, sliced

1 tbsp shredded basil leaves

1. Preheat the oven to 180°C (350°F/gas mark 4).

2. Bring a large pan of water to the boil and cook the pasta for 10 minutes.

3. Meanwhile, heat the olive oil in a frying pan and cook the onion for 2–3 minutes.

4. Add the mushrooms and sugar snap peas to the onion, then add a splash of water to steam-fry. Cook for 3–4 minutes, stirring occasionally.

5. Drain the pasta and return to the pan. Add the spinach and stir gently to wilt the spinach.

6. Add the mushroom and sugar snap pea mixture along with the soft cheese and cottage cheese. Stir well to mix, then season.

7. Pour the pasta into an ovenproof dish and top with the tomato slices. Bake in the oven for 15–20 minutes.

8. Sprinkle on the basil leaves to serve.

This dish is great for children. Serve it with a side salad if you want to add extra vegetables to your meal. For some variety, you can swap any of the vegetables for another of your choice – experiment with your favourites.

Grilled chicken with mash

Serves 4

8 chicken thighs with skin and bone (or a mixture of thighs and legs)

Juice of 1 lemon

3 tsp dried rosemary

Salt and pepper

900 g potatoes, peeled and cut into chunks

4 tbsp milk

2 tsp olive oil

Broccoli, steamed

1. Pre-heat the grill. Line a roasting tray with tin foil and place the chicken skin-side down on the foil. Squeeze half of the lemon over the chicken, then add half of the rosemary, and season. Grill for 15–20 minutes.

2. Boil the potatoes until soft (approx. 15–20 minutes). While the potatoes are cooking, turn over the chicken and squeeze over the remaining lemon. Sprinkle on the remaining rosemary and season, then grill for a further 15 minutes.

3. Mash the potatoes with the milk, olive oil and season lightly.

4. Serve the chicken with the mash and steamed broccoli.

Tuna pasta

Serves 4

200 g wholewheat pasta

1 tbsp extra-virgin olive oil

1 onion, peeled and chopped

1 garlic clove, peeled and finely chopped

400 g can chopped tomatoes

1 tbsp tomato purée

125 g sweetcorn (no added sugar or salt)

200 g can tuna (in water or brine), drained and flaked

1 tsp dried basil

Salt and freshly ground black pepper

1. Cook the pasta according to the directions on the packet.

2. Meanwhile, heat the olive oil in a large non-stick frying pan. Add the onion, garlic and tomatoes, and cook until the onion is soft.

3. Stir in the tomato purée and sweetcorn and cook for 5 minutes.

4. Add the tuna and basil, and heat through.

5. Stir the sweetcorn and tuna sauce into the pasta, season to taste and serve immediately.

Meal planning

These next few recipes are great for all the family. They're easy to make, so try cooking a batch at the weekend and freezing portions so you'll always have a dinner handy in the freezer. They'll keep in the fridge for a couple of days too.

Coconut chicken curry

Serves 4

1 ½ tbsp olive oil

1 onion, peeled and chopped

1 garlic clove, peeled and finely chopped

1 red chilli, finely chopped (optional)

4 skinless chicken breasts, cubed

200 ml light coconut milk

200 ml chicken stock

2 tbsp mild curry paste (Korma works well)

1 tbsp tomato purée

1 tbsp garam masala (optional)

200 g frozen peas

1 small sweet potato (or butternut squash), peeled and cut into bite-size chunks

Salt and freshly ground black pepper

Mix of cooked brown and white rice (50 g dry rice per person)

1. Heat the oil in a wok or frying pan and sauté the onion and garlic until soft. Add the chilli (if using).

2. Add the chicken and sauté for 4 minutes or until the meat is white all over.

3. Add the coconut milk and stock. Stir in the curry paste, tomato purée and garam masala (if using). Add the frozen peas and sweet potato. Simmer on a low heat until the sweet potato is soft (about 25 minutes). Season to taste.

4. Serve with a mix of brown and white rice cooked together (50 g dry rice per person).

Spaghetti bolognese

Serves 4

2 tbsp olive oil

1 large onion, peeled and finely chopped

½ stick celery, finely chopped

2 small garlic cloves, peeled and finely chopped

1 red pepper, finely chopped

400 g lean minced beef

400 g can chopped tomatoes

100 ml chicken, vegetable or beef stock

3 tbsp tomato purée

½ tsp dried thyme

½ tsp dried oregano

½ tsp dried basil

Salt and freshly ground black pepper

280 g wholewheat spaghetti

1. Heat the oil in a saucepan and sauté the onion and celery over a low heat for about 5 minutes, stirring occasionally until softened.

2. Add the garlic and pepper and cook for 5 minutes.

3. Add the minced beef and stir to break up. Cook until all the meat is browned (about 5–10 minutes).

4. Add the tomatoes, stock, tomato puree and herbs. Add a pinch of salt and pepper, to taste. Cover and cook over a low heat for about 25 minutes.

5. Meanwhile, cook the spaghetti according to the packet instructions. Drain and serve with the Bolognese sauce.

Chilli con carne

Serves 4

1½ tbsp olive oil

1 large onion, peeled and finely chopped

2 garlic cloves, peeled and finely chopped

1 small red chilli, deseeded and finely chopped, or 1 tsp dried chilli flakes

1 red pepper, deseeded and finely chopped

1 green pepper, deseeded and finely chopped

400 g extra-lean beef mince

Pinch of salt and freshly ground black pepper

1 tsp dried thyme

½ tsp paprika

1 bay leaf

1 tsp fennel seeds

½ tsp ground cinnamon

1 tsp chilli powder (mild or medium)

400 g can chopped tomatoes

½ tbsp Worcestershire sauce

400 g can kidney beans, drained and rinsed

150 ml vegetable stock

Mix of cooked brown and white rice (50 g dry rice per person)

1. Heat a large non-stick saucepan or casserole, and add the olive oil. Stir-fry the onion, garlic and chilli for 5 minutes, or until softened, adding a little water if necessary.

2. Add the red and green peppers and cook for 3–5 minutes.

3. Add the mince and stir-fry, breaking it up with a wooden spoon, for 10 minutes, or until it is browned all over. Season and add all the other ingredients.

3. Bring to the boil, then cover and simmer gently for 1 hour, stirring occasionally.

4. Remove the bay leaf and serve with a mix of brown and white rice.

Fish pie

Serves 4

900 g potatoes, peeled and chopped

225 g salmon fillet

225 g undyed smoked haddock (cod or other white fish fillet also works well)

150 ml semi-skimmed milk

2 tsp olive oil

200 g mushrooms, chopped

1 onion, peeled and finely chopped

100 g fresh spinach

6 tbsp low-fat fromage frais

3 tbsp mix of dill and flat-leaf parsley, chopped

Salt and black pepper

1. Preheat the oven to 200°C (400°F/gas mark 6).

2. Boil the potatoes until tender (approx. 15–20 minutes).

3. Place the fish and milk in a small pan and simmer for 4–5 minutes until the fish is just cooked. Drain, reserving the milk. Flake the fish into large chunks.

4. Heat the olive oil in a pan, add the mushrooms, onion and spinach, and cook for 4–5 minutes until the spinach has wilted.

5. Add the fish and fromage frais, stir well to combine and simmer for 1–2 minutes before stirring in the herbs and seasoning. Transfer to a shallow dish.

6. Drain the potatoes and mash with 100 ml of the reserved milk. Season and spoon over the fish.

7. Place in the oven and cook for 10 minutes, until the potato topping is bubbling and golden.

7. Serve with steamed broccoli and peas.

Weekend treats

These recipes are ready in an hour, so they're great for weekends or when you have a little more time.

Pesto chicken and roasted vegetables

Serves 4

900 g new potatoes

2 tbsp olive oil

4 boneless and skinless chicken breasts

4 tbsp basil pesto

3 medium courgettes, sliced

2 red onions, peeled and chopped

1 red or yellow pepper, deseeded and chopped

Salt and freshly ground black pepper

1. Preheat the oven to 200°C (400°F/gas mark 6).

2. Chop the potatoes into 2-cm chunks, keeping the skin on. Place in a large roasting tin and drizzle over the olive oil. Roast in the oven for 15 minutes, until the potatoes begin to soften and turn golden.

3. Remove the roasting tin, scrape the potatoes if they're sticking to the bottom and carefully lay the chicken breasts among the potatoes.

4. Spread a quarter of the pesto over each breast. Pile the rest of the vegetables around the tin and season with salt and pepper.

5. Return to the oven and cook for a further 20–25 minutes, until cooked through.

5. Serve with a green salad or green vegetables.

Grilled spicy salmon with roast butternut squash

Serves 4

Olive oil spray

2 large butternut squashes
(approx 2.5 kg), peeled and cut
into large chunks

Salt and black pepper

2 tsp mild chilli powder

4 tsp cumin

1 tbsp soy sauce

4 skinned salmon fillets

Mixture of steamed green
vegetables (broccoli, sugar snap
peas and courgette)

1. Preheat the oven to 220°C
   (425°F/gas mark 7).

2. Spray a baking tray with olive oil
   spray and bake the squash with
   a little salt and pepper for 45
   minutes, or until soft. If you prefer
   mash, it can now be mashed.
   Keep warm.

3. Mix the chilli powder, cumin and
   soy sauce together, and rub into
   the salmon.

4. Preheat the grill to a high setting
   or heat a non-stick pan with 1
   teaspoon olive oil. Grill the salmon
   for 6–8 minutes (3–4 minutes on
   each side if using a pan).

5. Serve with the squash and steamed
   green vegetables.

The Gunning Family from Luton

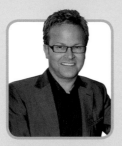

Steve visited the Gunnings from Luton.

'I'm about to meet three jelly-bellied jumbos whose lumbering lifestyle has sent their waistbands groaning and top buttons moaning …

'After a hard week at work Kim and Wayne can't wait to get home on a Friday to indulge in their favourite pastime – food. From Friday till Sunday they're constantly snacking their way through a house full of sweets and treats, and eating takeaways.

'Mum Sally's no better with her non-stop biscuit popping.

'This family barely get out of the house. Kim and Wayne have become old before their time and Sally doesn't have a man in her life. Oh no! She has a biscuit tin instead!

'Between them they're packing in 9,450 calories every day. That's more than enough food to sustain another fully grown man.'

The stats (after eight weeks)

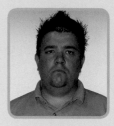

Son: **Wayne**
Age: **35**
Height: **5' 8"**
Start weight: **18 st 4 lb**
Now weighs: **15 st 4 lb**

Total weight loss: **3 st**

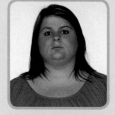

Fiancée: **Kim**
Age: **21**
Height: **5' 5"**
Start weight: **18 st 1 lb**
Now weighs: **15 st 10 lb**

Total weight loss: **2 st 5 lb**

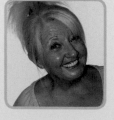

Mum: **Sally**
Age: **59**
Height: **5' 0"**
Start weight: **11 st 7 lb**
Now weighs: **10 st 4 lb**

Total weight loss: **1 st 3 lb**

Total family weight loss: **6 st 8 lb**

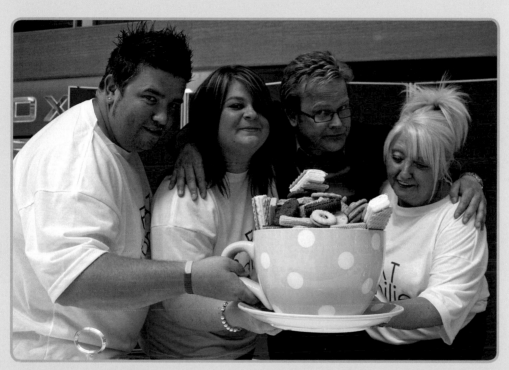

Main problem

Both Kim and Wayne work full-time – Kim for a property management company and Wayne as a fabricator – and although Kim likes cooking, it was tempting to have a takeaway in the evenings. Weekends were one big feast of burgers, pizzas, kebabs and Chinese, from breakfast until dinner.

They ate huge meals in the evenings and did absolutely no exercise to work them off before bed. No wonder they felt tired and lacking in energy and sat in front of the TV all night!

Kim has been overweight since she was a child and had tried every sort of crash diet and diet club imaginable, but always put the weight back on.

Sally works nights as an auxiliary nurse caring for the terminally ill and found the topsy-turvy hours disturbed her eating patterns. She rarely ate proper meals and snacked on biscuits, cakes, doughnuts and sandwiches. During her time off, because she lives alone, she couldn't be bothered to cook meals. She admits that she's a fussy eater so couldn't face meat that had any fat or gristle on it, overloading on carbs instead. She had become quite depressed, sitting at home alone and not wanting to meet up with friends.

Main motivation

Kim and Wayne are engaged and Kim wants a proper wedding, with lovely photographs, a beach holiday where she can feel proud to wear a bikini without covering up with a sarong and, most of all, to have children without endangering her health and being a fat mum.

Kim says, 'My mum and my sister are very small and glam and my dad lost three stone recently because of his diabetes so I know that I shouldn't be this weight.'

Sally admits that she had become depressed by her weight gain. She had an operation two years ago

for which she managed to give up smoking after 43 years, but she piled on the weight instead. 'My confidence went, I stayed home and didn't go out, not even to visit my sister.'

And Wayne wanted to start looking and feeling better. He plays football a couple of times a week but got out breath easily.

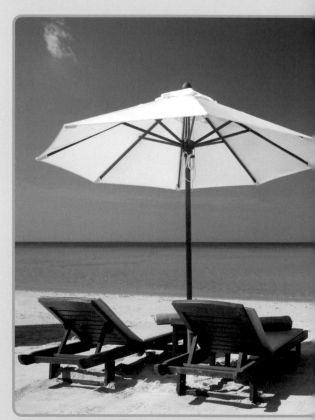

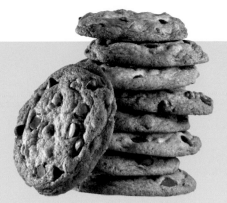

Typical day's food: Kim

Breakfast:	Nothing or a chocolate biscuit and crisps
11am:	Chocolate bar, diet cola, crinkle-cut potato chips
Lunch:	Sandwich/wrap, chocolate bar, crisps
Dinner:	2 chicken Kievs, large jacket potato with butter, vegetables or takeaway

Weekends:	Fast-food breakfast
Lunch:	Kebab, chips
Dinner:	Chinese takeaway, ice cream

Medical tests

We ran tests on the Gunnings and found:

Kim: had dangerously high blood pressure and high cholesterol, which could lead to heart problems. Over 50% of her body weight was fat. Kim has a slightly underactive thyroid that slowed her metabolism and she blamed it for her weight, but Professor McCarthy told her it just meant she had to work that bit harder to lose weight. At her age she had plenty of time to turn things around.

Wayne: although his blood pressure and cholesterol weren't too bad, he was carrying 44% of his body weight as fat, which meant he was increasing his risk of a stroke or heart attack.

Sally: was devastated to learn that in addition to her high blood pressure she was showing signs of liver damage. 'I broke down and cried. I had cancer when I was 22 and I think the drugs damaged my liver but this really scared me.'

Lifestyle changes

Kim and Wayne need to remind themselves that they are a young couple who should be out doing things instead of sitting in front of the TV. Wayne still plays football, but

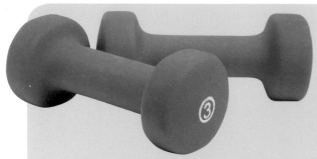

he's hampered by his weight. And Sally knows inside that she uses her eating as a comfort – but it's making her even more unhappy.

They needed to:

1. Drastically reduce their portion sizes
2. Cut out the chocolate – Kim ate chocolate every single day
3. Start walking instead of driving everywhere
4. Ban takeaways and start cooking from scratch
5. Stop stuffing themselves before bed

Exercise regime

Personal trainer Chris O'Hanlon took on the Gunnings and threw them in at the deep end so they would know from the start what was expected of them.

He took them to a field and made them jog around the edge of it!

They were given a treadmill at home and signed up to do three sessions with Chris each week, usually two in the gym and one outdoors, where they had to run around a field, do star jumps and squats. He also put them through a farmer's run – around the field ten times with weights in their hand, then a decreasing number of press-ups on each run followed by 50 lunges on each leg.

Chris said, 'I've put them through a very wide range of exercises: stability balls, squats, lunges, power walking, tricep presses, farmer's runs – Kim and Wayne are young enough to be able to take the pressure! To be honest, neither Kim nor Sally took to exercise that easily – I think they were used to giving up when the going got tough and there were a few tears along the way. But you can either start losing weight when you're young or you can start when you've had your first heart attack – the choice is yours.

'But once Kim started to see the results of all the hard work and got on the scales she turned a corner and got her nose to the grindstone. I think she is really motivated to lose more weight and keep going.

> Wayne: 'We had a day trip to the fair and I couldn't fit on one of the rides – it was so embarrassing.'

'Sally is older but she works very hard and doesn't moan – her big issue isn't exercise, it's about managing her eating.

'She was substituting meals with fruit and you can't mess around when you are doing intensive exercising. Jessica gave her a helping hand and I hope that she's getting the right balance now.

'Wayne is really on board – sometimes when he's working out I can see the pain on his face and how much of a struggle it is but he keeps pushing and the results are really worth it. Kim and Wayne can give each other a lot of support and I think it's harder for Sally being on her own, but if she can crack the eating she certainly can do the exercise.'

Sally said, 'I did find it difficult keeping up with people so much younger than me and I think when you work nights a lot your body never quite adjusts.'

Wayne, however, is enjoying the improved fitness. 'It was a bit of a shock at first but now Chris is pleased with my recovery rate and I'm into the press-ups. The blokes at the football

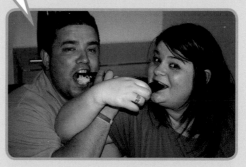

club have always called me by a nickname – Bubbles – now they're worried what to call me!'

Healthy eating

Jessica Wilson was worried that Kim and Wayne ate so much at night. Not only did they have a huge meal but they carried on the rest of the evening – Kim could eat a whole tube of Pringles after a full meal. And Sally wasn't eating proper food at all, just snacking on high-fat and sugary snacks with almost no nutritional value.

They were given portion control plates, as Kim and Wayne seemed to have no idea how much they were eating. A lot of food went in their mouths without them being aware of it.

Sally needed to plan ahead. Her breakfast consisted of a cup of tea and a pile of biscuits and when she was on the night shift her co-workers shared cakes and snacks all night. Her lifestyle was affecting her long-term health with signs of fatty liver.

All three of them needed to start eating fresh fruit and vegetables and to junk the high-fat takeaways. They also needed to be aware of what they ate – Sally would eat up to 15 biscuits for breakfast because she was just nibbling instead of having a proper meal. They never seemed to stop eating when they were full!

Jessica helped Sally with a meal plan for single people – it can be harder to eat healthily when you live alone. And she needed to build up the protein content of her meals.

Progress highs and lows

Kim found giving chocolate up the hardest part.

'I went to my mum's the other day and she had a Toblerone. I just smelled it and thought, I could eat this in 20 seconds – but then it would take an hour to burn it off! I think I've weaned myself off it now.

'My high point was finding an old skirt from Next that I used to wear – in a size 18. I was a 22 and I can wear this to work now!'

Sally hit a low point when one week she lost just one pound. 'I felt so disappointed. All that effort of watching what I was eating and then to lose just one pound – you think, shall I chuck it in? But we keep each other going. I don't want to let anyone else down.'

Wayne went to his uncle's barbecue a couple of weeks into the plan and found it hard not to stuff himself like he used to.

'I had a little nibble but was it worth it? Now I feel great because I bought myself a designer T-shirt ages ago that grew tighter and tighter until I had to stop wearing it. Now it's loose!'

The family says:

Kim: 'I used to feel happy when I ate a lot but then straight afterwards I would feel really low. I was

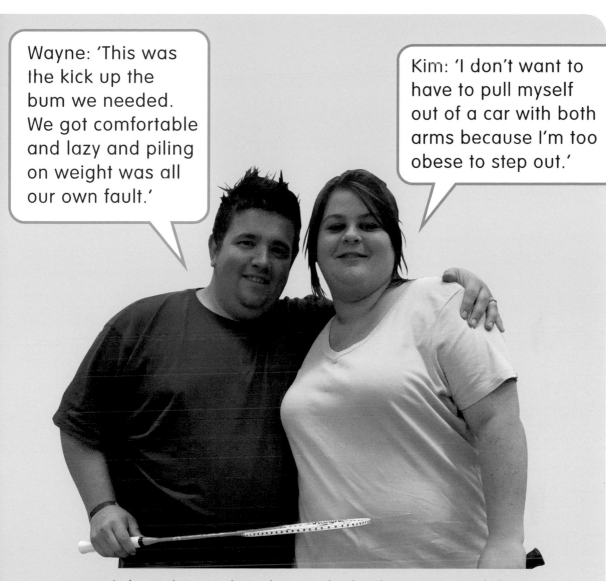

Wayne: 'This was the kick up the bum we needed. We got comfortable and lazy and piling on weight was all our own fault.'

Kim: 'I don't want to have to pull myself out of a car with both arms because I'm too obese to step out.'

paranoid about what people said about me, even though I seemed confident. I had no energy. When I was told at the medical that I wasn't just obese, I was *massively* obese, it was a real shock.

'Now I don't miss the old lifestyle at all. I love cooking and we can have some of our favourites, such as chilli con carne, but not in massive portions. I used to play badminton at school and now I've started playing again. When I go to the supermarket I park in the furthest space from the doors, I use the stairs, I carry my own shopping instead of expecting Wayne to do it.

'I feel so much happier and I've got lots of things to look forward to. I do get scared that maybe I'll drift back but unlike the diets I did in the past I've got Wayne and Sally's support and it's my whole life that's changed.'

Wayne: 'I was quite slim as a child and I realise just how lazy I'd got, piling on weight. We have healthy food now and it isn't boring – I've got into stir-fries and love a chicken and lime stir-fry with loads of vegetables. I used to drive to the local shop, which is literally two minutes away – I'd never do that now.

'And Kim and I had got so lazy, we'd just sit on the sofa and watch TV – it's nice to do more things together We've stuck on the fridge a picture Steve gave us of what we could look like in five years' time – we don't want to be facing that.

'This isn't like a diet and I feel so much more confident than before. Other people's comments mattered to us and now we know we're losing weight we feel better.'

Sally: 'I do not want to go back to being the depressed person who shut herself away and wouldn't even answer the phone. I know I get down if I don't lose weight every week but I keep going. I can't live on biscuits forever and I can prepare food for work – even a little baked potato to microwave.

'I always wore baggy clothes but as my confidence built up I started to wear better clothes. I wouldn't say it's easy but doing it as a family makes all the difference.'

The Gunning family's top tips

- Keep going. If you have a bad week, ask for help.

- Use smaller plates – use side plates so you can't pile food on the edges.

- Watch the alcohol – it's a waste of calories.

- Don't be tempted by cereal bars instead of breakfast – they're loaded with sugar.

- Don't switch on the TV until you've done some sort of exercise.

- Don't buy chocolate!

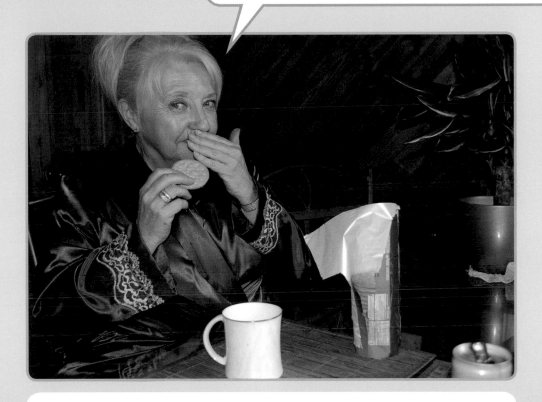

Sally: 'I never want to go back to shutting myself away because of how big I am.'

BISCUIT BONANZA

Sally's breakfast of up to 15 biscuits with a cup of tea was a total waste of 570 calories (38 per biscuit). For the same amount of calories she could have had:

Muesli (60 g portion) = 226 calories

AND wholemeal toast (2 slices) = 162 calories

AND 2 poached eggs = 148 calories

AND Flora light spread (8 g serving) = 28 calories

The Gunning family

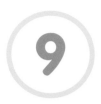

Exercise

As we said at the very beginning, this book is about changing your lifestyle, not just about losing weight. And one of the ways in which you will make a major change to your life – and help shed pounds at the same time – is to start becoming much more physically active than you are now.

Whether you work, are trying to find work or are at home bringing up children, the chances are that you feel tired by the end of the day. You slump in front of the TV, maybe with a beer or glass of wine, maybe with a takeaway because you're too tired to cook, or a packet of biscuits to snack on in front of a film.

You may have been very busy all day – but being busy isn't the same as being active and the tiredness you feel is probably more mental than physical.

If you've been working hard at a desk all day your head may be spinning but you may not actually have moved much at all. If you work in a shop, your feet and legs may ache from standing all day – but that's not the same as being physically active.

One of the great bonuses of getting fit is that you can actually do more and feel less tired.

Take an honest look at your day and see how much moving around you really do. Do you drive or take the bus to work or drive the kids to school? Take the lift up to your work floor? Send emails to people just across the other side of the room? Eat lunch at your desk or just pop into the canteen? When you get home do you walk around the block, take the dog out, go swimming with the kids?

Most us actually move an awful lot less than we think we do.

> **FACT**
> Inactive people are almost twice as likely to die from heart disease compared to active people.

TOP 10 REASONS FOR BECOMING MORE ACTIVE

1. Regular exercise can reduce high blood pressure and lower levels of 'bad' cholesterol.

2. Regular exercise can help reduce weight, which lowers the risk of type 2 diabetes, cardiovascular disease and strokes.

3. Certain exercise can build lean muscle tissue, which burns more calories whether you are active or resting.

4. Exercise has been shown to protect against colon cancer and breast cancer in women past the menopause.

5. Exercise can help improve mild depression.

6. Exercise can help slow down or even repair the loss of bone mass, and prevent osteoporosis.

7. Exercise helps tone your body, which will improve your shape as you lose weight.

8. Exercise can strengthen muscle groups that will help with bad backs, and can improve flexibility and balance.

9. Exercise can improve your digestion and help you to sleep better. Lack of sleep alters your hormone balance and can even cause you to put on weight.

10. Taking regular exercise will encourage your children to exercise and prevent them becoming obese.

Take the pedometer test

Why not actually count how many steps you take on a normal day? Unless you are in a very physically demanding job it's likely that you take far fewer steps than the recommended minimum of around 10,000 a day.

You can test this out yourself with a pedometer. A pedometer is simply a tiny counting device that you clip to your waistband that clocks up each step you take by detecting the motion of your hips as you put one leg in front of the other. There are many different sorts and price ranges on the market – some simply count steps whereas others can be adjusted to measure the length of your stride and therefore calculate how many kilometres or miles you have walked.

But a simple, basic pedometer costs as little as £10 and it's a great way of starting to monitor your fitness levels – you may be amazed by how many (or how few!) steps you actually take in a day.

Use it for three days, record each day's amount, add them together and then divide by three. This gives an average daily number of steps walked – because we all have days when we are more active than others. What you need to know is what your realistic daily fitness level is.

If you're into technology you'll find that lots of mobile phone companies now include pedometers in their products, some with GPS in case you get lost! And some Apple iPods and MP3 players also have a pedometer function so you can listen to music while you burn off those calories. Could they make it any easier to get started?

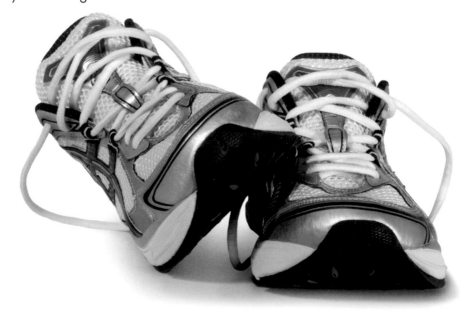

If you find that you're only walking about 3,000 or 4,000 steps a day, you'll realise just how much more you need to do before you're even at the baseline of getting fit!

Find what you like doing

The most important thing about taking up a more active life is to find an activity you enjoy. Some love running, out on their own in all weathers, improving their times. For others this is their idea of hell but doing a dance exercise class with friends is as good as a night out. If you don't enjoy your chosen exercise, the chances are you won't keep it up.

You don't have to join a gym or invest in expensive outfits or equipment – you can simply walk the dog for an hour a day or go for a jog around the park.

Swimming is another great form of exercise that builds lean muscle tissue and stamina. It's not as intensive a weight-loss exercise but it supports your joints and tightens your abdominals – and you're never too old to go swimming.

Russell Byham, who got the Huzzey family off their bottoms, says:

REMEMBER!
You should always check with your doctor before taking up any new form of exercise, especially if you suffer from high blood pressure, heart problems or have any other health concerns.

Always have proper instruction from a qualified trainer before using any gym equipment or weights.

'If exercise is going to become a habit it must be enjoyable. There's something out there for everyone and it's down to the stage in life they're at and whether they like doing it alone or with other people.'

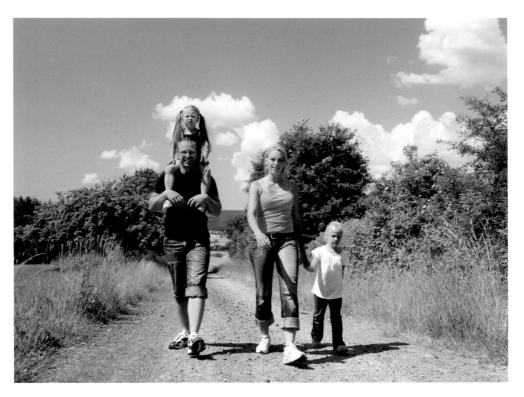

Walking for everyone

Even if you've never done any exercise before, you can start walking more. Walking has a huge number of benefits – for your health, weight and social life.

For a start, it's completely free, you can do it anywhere and you don't need expensive equipment – although you do need a good pair of trainers or walking shoes that offer support, cushioning and flexibility.

You can walk on your own, with friends or with a dog – and there are plenty of people willing to lend you their friendly mutt on a cold winter's day! (If you live alone, walking a dog is a fantastic way of making friends!)

It's good for your heart and cardiovascular system, especially if you keep up a decent pace and swing your arms. It's good for your legs, tones up your bottom and lifts your spirits.

Start by walking to the local shop instead of driving, or walking to collect the kids from school. It might only take ten minutes but it's ten minutes you weren't doing last week. Try to keep up a pace where you can chat to a friend without getting breathless but you're putting in some effort – swing your arms a bit faster and your legs will speed up to keep pace.

Aim to increase the number of steps you take by 1,000 a day above your average starting total – it doesn't all have to be done in one go but you need to make progress week by week in order to see any fitness benefits. It should be quite easy to build 10,000 steps a day into your new routine – but this is only a guideline, you don't have to stop here!

It's hard to imagine when you first start, but a brisk walk is one of the first activities where you will notice your energy levels improve. Then you can progress to include other sorts of exercise in your life that will strengthen and tone muscles, and burn fat. A vigorous walk can burn up to 195 calories in 30 minutes (depending on your weight).

Interval training

Interval training is a good thing to introduce once you've been walking briskly for further distances for around six to eight weeks. Interval training means you combine your normal brisk walking pace with short, sharp bursts of increased activity – these 'supercharge' your metabolic rate so you burn fat faster.

These periods of increased activity can be as short as 15 seconds, although as you get fitter you'll make the bursts longer. If you can teach yourself a good interval training routine, you'll find it can burn more fat in a shorter period of exercise as it's very efficient.

Set yourself little distances where you suddenly push yourself a bit harder, almost a jog, for anything from 15 to 60 seconds. Once your body is used to walking at a decent speed it needs to work harder, and interval training, in which you change the pace for brief periods, increases your consumption of energy and your ability to lose fat.

If you're walking on the streets, have a quick burst of speed between two lampposts or if you're in a park, run or jog between two trees.

And once you've got it going with a regular rhythm, pushing yourself closer to your maximum heart rate, you'll find you need to do it for shorter periods to achieve the same fitness result.

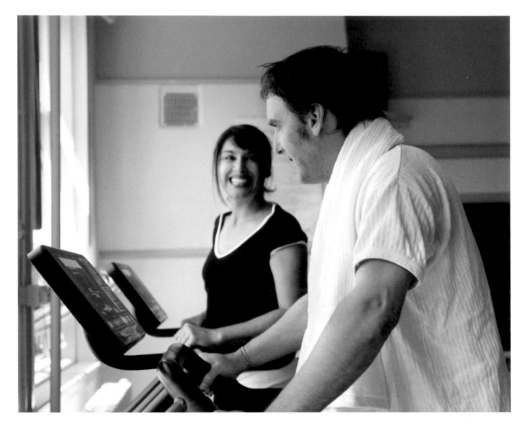

Walking as a family also gives you a chance to talk and support each other as you lose weight and change your habits. If you haven't anyone to walk with, check on the internet for walking clubs in your area – or start one of your own!

MONITORING YOUR HEART RATE

Taking exercise can make your heart more efficient, so that it doesn't have to work as hard to pump blood around your body. As you get fitter you will notice your heart rate changes and you can monitor the number of times it beats per minute (take your pulse) to judge how hard you should be exercising. Your different heart rates are as follows:

- Resting heart rate: This is the number of times per minute your heart beats when you are completely rested. The fitter you are, the fewer beats your heart has to make to send blood around the body. The average person's resting heart rate is in the low 70s. Some ultra-fit athletes have resting rates in the low 40s! The best time to take this is when you first wake up in the morning. Take it each day for three days to get the average. Place your index and middle fingers over the artery running through the inside of your wrist and press very gently. You should feel the blood pumping under your fingers. Count the beats for one minute to get your heart rate.

- Maximum heart rate: This is the highest number of times your heart can pump per minute when you are exercising. It is determined by age, sex and fitness levels and to measure it accurately you should use a specialised machine on a treadmill.

- Recovery heart rate: This is the rate at which your heart slows down after a period of intense exercise – the fitter you are, the faster your heart should return to normal. For example, if you exercise for 30 minutes at 155 beats per minute, then stop and take your heart rate after two minutes rest, it may have come down to something like 95.

WORKING OUT YOUR HEART RATE

To monitor how hard your body is working when you exercise you need to work out what your ideal heart rate work range is. You do this by first working out what your maximum heart rate is by subtracting your age from 220. This is a rough equation but gives an idea of how intensively your heart should be working.

So if you are aged 30, your maximum heart rate will be:

For a man: 220–30 = 190 beats per minute

For a woman: 226–30 = 196 beats per minute

When you are exercising safely but effectively you need to be working at a percentage of your maximum heart rate. To start burning fat, you need to work at 60–70% of your maximum heart rate. To improve your cardiovascular fitness you need to work at 70–80% of your maximum heart rate. Measure how long it takes for your heart rate to come back down to normal. This is a good indication of how fit you are – a rough guide to how quickly it should return to normal is to check your pulse immediately after you stop exercising then again after one minute. It should have slowed by around 12 beats per minute.

Warming up

Whatever your fitness levels or chosen exercise, some rules apply to everyone. And the first is that it is very important to warm up properly before starting any form of exercise. Even professional footballers do a jog up and down the touchline and a few stretches before they go on as substitutes, and they haven't spent all day in front of a computer or sitting in front of the TV.

Warm-up exercises are gentle movements that literally warm up the muscles and increase their blood flow, bringing them more oxygen, so you are less likely to injure yourself. Warm muscles are more flexible and less likely to cramp or strain.

About ten minutes is a good warming-up period for most people and should raise your heart rate a bit without making it pump as hard as it should during the exercise programme itself.

If you're very unfit and coming to exercise for the first time, you should warm up for as long as 15 minutes.

Opinion is divided on whether you should stretch after a warm-up and before exercising, or just afterwards when you are very warm – but never stretch cold muscles. If you stretch after a warm-up, it should be gentle.

Try these warm-up exercises

- Start walking up and down the room or on the spot, swinging your arms to work your upper body. March, with your knees lifting up a bit higher and your arms raised above your head, to make your heart pump that bit harder.
- Shake out your hands and arms loosely, and shake your lower leg loose from the ankle.

- Reach from side to side above your head to get your waist moving.

- Step to the side and back – try to get moving in all directions.

- If you're in the gym this is a good time to get on the bike and cycle for ten minutes, or do a bit of walking on the treadmill at an even pace.

- At home, you could walk up and down the stairs six times.

Professional trainers will tell you that you should warm up the muscles specifically being used for each activity you are about to do – for instance, running uses different muscles from the rowing machine – but for beginners it's important to remember that you're getting your body prepared for moving about – and it isn't used to it!

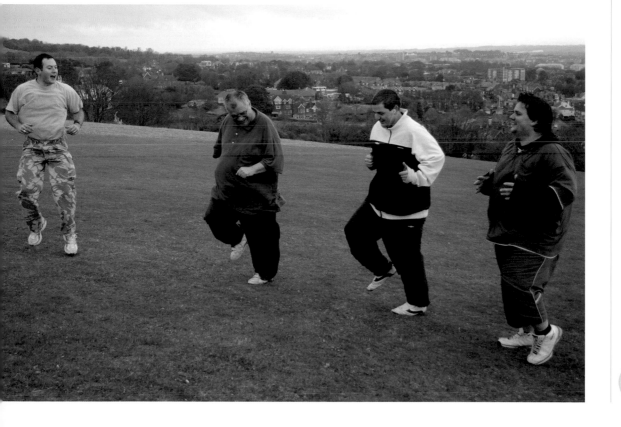

Cool down

After a workout of any sort, or even a long walk, it's important to gradually slow down rather than stop suddenly – and to give those hard-working muscles a bit of a stretch. This helps to relieve the build-up of lactic acid in the muscles, which causes cramps, and gives your heart a chance to adjust to the reduced effort you are making.

   You also need to make sure you aren't dehydrated so you may want to drink some water.

   On the treadmill or cross trainer you should slow gradually to a gentle walk and do that for at least two minutes.

   Stretching is a good way to cool down, and after exercise it's easier because your muscles are looser.

Calf stretch

Stand with your feet a natural stride apart, right leg in front of the left. Bend your right knee slightly and gently transfer the weight onto this leg while keeping the heel of the left leg on the ground. The stretch will be felt down the back of the left calf. Hold this for around 20 seconds – you may feel it tighten after about six seconds but it will then relax. Repeat on the other leg.

   Another good calf stretch is to stand on a low step,

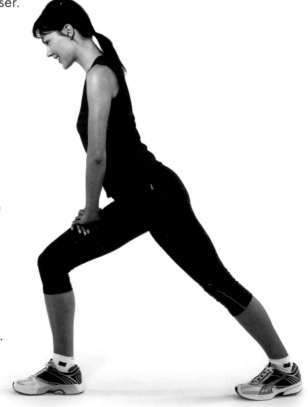

balancing on the front half of your foot, with both your heels hanging back over the step. Drop your heels down as far as you can so that you can feel a stretch down the back of your calf – this is a good one to do on the stairs if you exercise at home.

Thigh stretch

Stand with your feet parallel and knees close together. Bend one leg back and, holding the ankle with your hand, pull it in gently towards your buttock. Keeping your knees close together and your hips slightly pushed forward (don't bend forward from the waist), pull your ankle into your bottom as firmly as you can and hold for 15 to 20 seconds. You should feel a gentle pull down the whole of your front thigh. Swap legs and repeat.

If you find it hard to balance, you can do this on a gym mat or a carpet. Lie on your side, propping up your upper-body weight on a bent elbow, forearm flat to the floor. Bend your upper-leg knee and pull the ankle back in the same way. Roll over onto your other side and repeat for the other leg.

Hamstring stretch

Your hamstrings are the muscles that run down the back of the thigh. Most people who don't exercise and stretch regularly have very tight hamstrings.

Lift your leg and rest the heel on a bench or low flat surface (a coffee table will do), keeping your leg straight and your toes pointing straight up. Bend your back leg and, keeping your back straight, slide your hands down the straight leg towards your toes. If you're flexible, you can hold onto your upturned foot and try to stretch your toes back. You should feel a stretch right down the back of the thigh. Hold for 15 to 20 seconds until the thigh relaxes.

Shoulder stretches

Anyone who works on a computer or does a lot of driving will suffer from stiff, tight shoulders. These exercises help to loosen and mobilise the shoulder joints.

1. Lift both arms above your head. Bend one arm from the elbow and use the other hand to hold that elbow and gently guide the forearm down the middle of your back. Don't press on the elbow – the pressure should be light but firm. Hold for the stretch. Repeat with the other arm. This is good for shoulders and the triceps muscle (the one that runs along the back of your upper arm).

2. Link your hands behind your back, pulling your arms out as straight as you can. Gently pull back your arms, lifting them slightly. You should feel a pull across the front of your shoulders. Don't lean forward. This is an excellent exercise for helping to improve your posture if you are very round-shouldered.

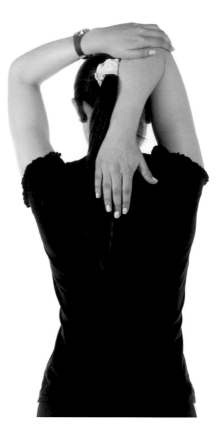

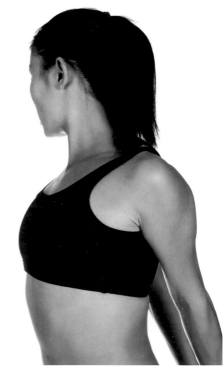

What's the right exercise for you?

Running/treadmill

Running is a great exercise for burning fat, improving your cardiovascular health, developing lean muscle and lifting your spirits. However, it isn't for everyone and if you find it boring, or find the repeated stress it puts on your knee or hip joints causes you problems, then don't do it. There are plenty of other exercises out there.

But if you do take up running, be warned – it can become addictive! Runners love nothing more than improving their times so if you have a bit of a competitive spirit, you may find this is the sport for you.

You can run outdoors or on a treadmill in the gym – it depends entirely on what fits in with your routine. Or get a treadmill at home, if you have space somewhere, and you can run all year round without worrying about the weather!

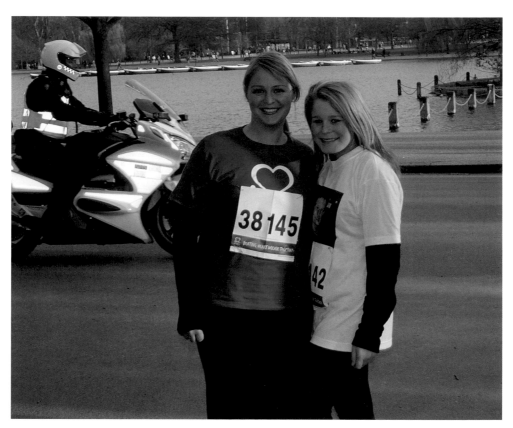

It's important to get the right pair of shoes if you are going to run regularly – a specialist sports shoe shop salesperson will look at your feet and may ask you to run on a mini-treadmill so they can see whether you roll your feet in or out when you run. But running shoes can be expensive so make sure this is the sport for you before you splash out on the gear.

Running with a partner or a couple of friends is a great way to maintain your interest and there are running clubs across the country – look them up on the internet. Here are some tips to get you started:

1. Start slow. You're not going to become an Olympic runner overnight. Start by jogging, keeping a pace that lets you talk but pushes you sufficiently to make your heart beat faster and bring you out in a bit of a sweat.

Use the interval-training techniques described on page 163 to go for short bursts of speed – then slow back down to a jog. If you have to stop for any reason (a level crossing, a busy road), keep jogging on the spot – the object is to keep your heart rate up and build some stamina.

When you progress to running (always after a good warm-up) you'll probably find you have to keep stopping – just keep walking/jogging and when you get a second wind, start running slowly a bit more.

2. Relax. Your body should be loose, not tense, with your arms swinging quite naturally at your side. Try not to lean forwards or backwards as this puts strain on your knees, and keep yourself as tall as possible. You shouldn't be hunched over for breath.

3. Don't be too ambitious. Stay on the flat, start with a jog and let your own pace develop over weeks. You will burn around 100 calories a mile to start off with, so you might want to combine it with a bit of strength training.

4. Enjoy it. This is supposed to be something you do for pleasure, so try to find places to run that will be uplifting. But even if you run around an industrial estate, listen to music on your iPod or think positive thoughts!

Gym work

If you can afford it, joining a gym gives you the chance to use a lot more equipment, maybe also a swimming pool, and there should be qualified staff to teach you how to use the machines safely and with the correct techniques.

Local authority gyms are usually a lot cheaper than private gyms and they may well have special rates for families or concessions you can take advantage of. They usually run aerobic, dance or kick-boxing classes and circuit training too, so that even if you don't want to become a gym bunny it's worth the fee.

Cross trainer

Using a cross trainer, sometimes known as an elliptical machine, is an excellent way of getting good cardiovascular exercise using your arms and legs, without the impact on your joints that you receive when jogging or running.

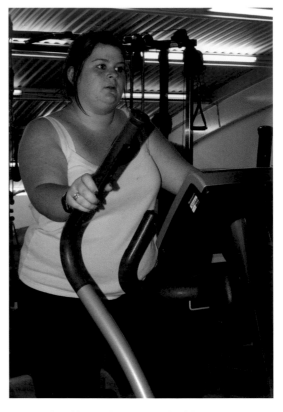

This type of exercise strengthens and builds your lower legs (try to keep your heels down on the footplate – it helps to stretch out the calves) and is good for the very overweight as it lessens any strain on the knees, hips and back.

You can vary the intensity of your session and, although you probably won't burn as many calories as when you run or row, you will be getting a good workout. And it's a weight-bearing exercise, despite the low impact, so is good for building bone strength.

Using your arms to push/pull the hand grips increases the cardiovascular effectiveness, but some people prefer to use just the leg plates, which can increase speed and also helps to develop your core muscles (the ones around your abdomen), which can relieve strain on your back.

Rowing machine

Some people worry that a rowing machine will be bad for their back but in fact, rowing with the right technique can strengthen the muscles that support your back. Like all gym equipment, it should only be used after instruction by a properly qualified instructor. Used in the right way, a rowing machine is an excellent low-impact cardiovascular activity, and it exercises all parts of your body.

It improves posture, strengthens core muscles and burns lots of calories. So if you can, it's a good one to build into your weekly exercise routine.

Weights

Forget Arnold Schwarzenegger – using weights isn't about building up bulging muscles, it's about building up strength so your muscles perform better. Using weights can improve your

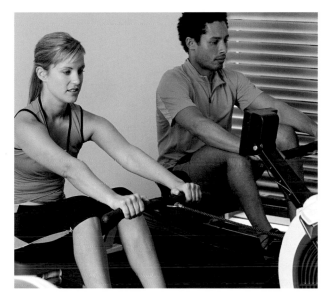

bone density and protect against the loss of muscle mass as you get older.

Ideally, you should combine some cardiovascular, fat-burning exercise with some weight-based exercises. As you develop more muscle tissue, your metabolism has to work a bit harder to feed it – you'll actually burn around 50 more calories every day for every pound of muscle you put on – that means you're burning more calories even while you watch TV!

And although muscle tissue is denser than fat and therefore weighs more by volume (a square inch of muscle is heavier than a square inch of fat) – that doesn't mean you will put on weight overall. As you lose fat and convert it to muscle you may see a little slow-down or reach that disheartening plateau where your weight appears to be stuck, but look at how differently your clothes hang on your newly emerging waist or how your upper arms wobble less!

Including weight training into your exercise routine can help with type 2 diabetes and high blood pressure, and is a nice change of pace from the higher-intensity cardiovascular activity.

It doesn't take long either – a couple of 20-minute sessions a week will start to transform that flab into muscle – and you can do it at home in front of the TV!

Try this now. Take two large cans of baked beans and do some bicep curls. Standing up, hold the tins in your hands and let your arms rest naturally down by your side, with your knees slightly bent. Bending from the elbows but keeping the elbows close into your waist, pull up your hands smoothly towards your shoulders and slightly twist them outwards as you do so, so that your palms face your shoulders. Breathe out as you raise your arms. Do this 20 times and then rest. You'll feel the difference those little weights make.

You can also do this by raising your arms away from your sides, stopping when they reach shoulder level. Keep your knees slightly bent and breathe out as you raise your arms. Of course, as you get stronger you'll find the baked bean cans too light, but we all have to start somewhere!

Circuit training

Circuit training is designed to maximise the number of muscle groups you use in order to build stamina, strength and flexibility.

Basically, it's a planned circuit of different exercises that you repeat a certain number of times each before you move from one exercise to the next – with a small break in between. You have a slightly longer rest at the end of the circuit before beginning the cycle again. You should try to vary the muscle groups you use in each exercise so that you rest them – so, for instance, don't do upper-body exercises one after the other. It sounds complicated – but it can be fun and is also a good way of measuring your progress.

A trainer at your local gym can design a circuit for you that will be well balanced and suited to your current level of fitness. You might use things like fitness balls, wobble boards, benches, weights and ropes. However, it is possible to devise a sort of circuit at home. For example, after your ten-minute warm-up you might do:

• 20 squats: stand with your feet hip-width apart and slowly bend your knees, lowering your hips towards the floor, as if sitting back into a chair. Keep your back straight and stomach in. Don't lower your knees more than 90 degrees – your thighs should be parallel with the ground.

- 20 press-ups: lie face-down on the floor with your hands slightly wider than shoulder width, bend your legs from the knee back towards your bottom and cross your ankles. Then press up with your arms, keeping your knees to the floor.

- 30 seconds of lunges (each leg): split your legs, placing one in front and one behind. Bend slowly from the knees, lowering your body until both knees are at 90 degrees. Push back from the feet into your starting position.

- 15 shoulder presses: stand up straight. Using a dumbbell (or large can of beans), hold the weight at shoulder-height, with your palms facing forward. Breathe out, pull in your abdominal muscles and slowly push your arm straight up overhead, making sure not to arch your back.

- 20 seconds of side-leg raises (each leg): stand straight, feet slightly apart, pull in your abdominal muscles and slowly lift your right leg out to the side, keeping your back straight. Hold for a couple of seconds before slowly lowering.

- 20 step-ups (each leg): keeping your back straight and relaxed, step onto a block with your right foot and bring the left up to meet it. Step back down, leading again with your right foot. You can keep leading with your right for ten steps then lead with the left for ten, or you can alternate each time.

- 25 abdominal crunches: lie down on your back, hands behind your head, with your knees bent and feet flat on the floor. As you breathe out, contract your abdominal muscles, so your lower back flattens against the floor, and slowly bring your shoulder blades a couple of inches off the floor. Hold this for a couple of seconds before lowering almost to the floor while you breathe in.

- 30 seconds of skipping with a rope.

... and so on, rotating the parts of your body you are working. You should see a professional trainer to learn how to do all of these exercises properly before trying them at home so you don't injure yourself.

Exercise

Dave Coard trained the Haddrell family and taught them a circuit-training exercise to do in their garden, using whatever equipment they could improvise.

He says, 'It's the combination of exercises that make a difference. Sarah was determined she couldn't do press-ups but you start by pushing yourself away from the wall to build up a bit of strength and in the end she could do them.'

A good thing about circuit training is that you can see your strengths and weaknesses and what you need to work on most. Even if you stop for a breather, it's important to keep moving around. Bear in mind that if you start out very overweight it's best to avoid high-impact exercise and concentrate on getting your weight down first.

Home gym

Your house is full of things that can be used to help you exercise, especially if you're a beginner – you don't need to spend lots of money at a gym.

- If you have a set of stairs, then climb up and down them six times to warm up.

- Marching up and down to some music gets your heart rate up – keep your arms swinging!

- Raid the kids' toybox for a skipping rope – never forget the old-fashioned hula-hoop – or try games like Wii Fit or a dance mat.

- A cheap bat and ball set will at least get you moving around in the park or the garden – not everything has to be formal exercise.

Keep reminding yourself that every five minutes you spend moving and away from the TV builds towards your daily exercise target.

Swimming

Swimming is one of those hobbies that will last you a lifetime and do you nothing but good. One of the great advantages of swimming is that the water supports your joints so they don't take the shock of impact as they can do when running or jogging. And, as trainer Russel Byham says, 'You can't hide your fitness in a swimming pool – you stop swimming – you sink!'

It's good cardiovascular exercise, as long as you put in a bit of effort, and tones abdominal, leg and shoulder muscles beautifully.

Swimming doesn't burn as many calories as more intensive exercise, but it depends on the stroke and the effort you put in. A fast front crawl can burn

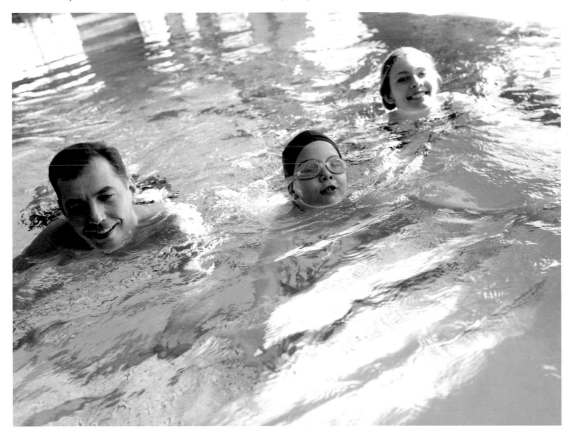

100 calories in 10 minutes, for example, whereas a breaststroke may only burn 60. But you're more likely to swim longer doing breaststroke, so the benefits could even out. Be careful not to stretch your neck up too far when swimming breaststroke, however, as you could strain it, and if you have knee problems check whether the breaststroke kick could make them worse.

Swimming is a good choice of exercise for the very overweight, wonderful for doing with children and can even be done safely while pregnant.

And you don't have to flog up and down the training pool for 50 lengths. Do 20 minutes' lane swimming then have some fun – diving (if you're allowed), going down the flumes and slides (up all those steps – good!), playing with the kids or just walking around against the water pressure.

When you're on holiday make the most of sea swimming – resisting the current or leaping in and out of the waves increases your energy expenditure.

If you can't swim, then look up adult classes at your local pool. You'll be amazed how quickly you become water-confident and, if you're a parent, it will set a great example to your children.

Aquaerobics

This is a really good all-round exercise – it improves the cardiovascular system, tones up the muscles, supports the joints as you work – and is great fun.

It's basically an exercise class that takes place in the shallow water of a swimming pool – usually around chest- or armpit-height. The exercises are a combination of ones you'd find in an aerobics class: jumping jacks, running on the spot, knee lifts, stretching, bum toning, etc.

One way in which aquaerobics scores highly is that the density of the water means it provides 12 times the resistance of air pressure, so your muscles are having to work 12 times as hard as they would doing the same exercises on land.

But because about 90% of your body is supported by the water, there's less strain on your joints and back – so it's a good option for people who worry about knee stress or back strain.

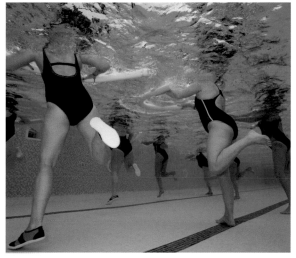

An aquaerobics class is slower than a gym-based one, however, and you won't burn as many calories as you would do on land – a 30-minute class could use around 300 calories – but if you combine it with other more intensive fat-burning exercises it will help to tone you up as the fat melts away. Why not get there a bit earlier and have a lane swim for 20 minutes first? Get a group of your friends to go with you and it becomes a fun evening out!

Cycling

The high level of traffic on our roads nowadays puts many people off outdoor cycling, which is a shame as it's a great form of everyday exercise that can be built into your normal life. Cycling to work or on light shopping trips also frees you from the expense and problems of parking!

You can use a bike in the gym, which is great for cardiovascular health and lower-body strength, but it's a shame not to take advantage of the health benefits of cycling outdoors. It's particularly good for very overweight people, as the saddle takes the strain of about 70% of your body weight, relieving pressure on the hip and knee joints.

The intensity at which you cycle and your age and body weight affect how many calories you burn. But someone who weighs around 12.5 stone will burn more than 650 calories in an hour's bike ride – and tone up the leg and bum muscles.

It's also a really good family day out and encourages the children to come away from the computer.

Lots of big parks and recreation areas have bike-hire stations, where you can hire tandems and covered baby buggies you tow behind the bikes! They're making it as easy as they can to get you all out there.

Remember to put a few bottles of water and some healthy snacks in a backpack so you can stop when the little ones need a break.

And everyone should wear a helmet – lead by example. No, they don't always look cool for teenagers, but it's a lot cooler than ending up with a fractured skull.

Skipping

You can get a really good workout by skipping. No, it's not girlie – it's a favourite exercise for boxers ... Done at speed it can burn up to 320 calories in 30 minutes. It improves the cardiovascular system, increases agility, coordination and balance, and tones legs, abdominals, back, chest and shoulders. The impact on the joints is medium, so it's a good choice for most people and helps to build bone mass.

The British Rope Skipping Association (yes, there is one!) claims that 10 minutes skipping can have the same health benefits as a 45-minute run, so here are some skipping tips:

- Stick on some music and start reasonably quickly so the rope doesn't tangle.

- Try to alternate your starting foot to keep your effort balanced. Skipping is a great exercise to alternate with strength training.

- You can buy fancy ropes that calculate how many calories you've burned but you can also use a length of old washing line – so no budget excuses!

- Ask someone old enough to remember to teach you playground skipping rhymes – then you can liven it up by doing it with friends!

- Another version is the ankle skipper – a loop that fits around your ankle with a rope attached to it and a ball at the end of it – which you whip around in a circular motion as you skip over it. It's much harder than it looks and you can work up quite a sweat.

Dance

At heart, we all want to be able to dance. Ever watched guests at a wedding after a few glasses of bubbly?

And we can, in the privacy of our own homes, stick on a selection of dance music and just let rip. It'll get you moving and improve your mood no end. It's also a great way of embarrassing teenagers in front of their friends!

But if you want something more formal, take a dance exercise class. Not only is it fun and sociable, but it's brilliantly healthy.

Dancers always warm up with some light exercise to improve flexibility. It's a very effective way of extending muscle mass to give a longer, leaner look. It builds muscle strength as the muscles work to lift and twist your body weight and it also builds stamina, increasing your heart rate and cardiovascular endurance.

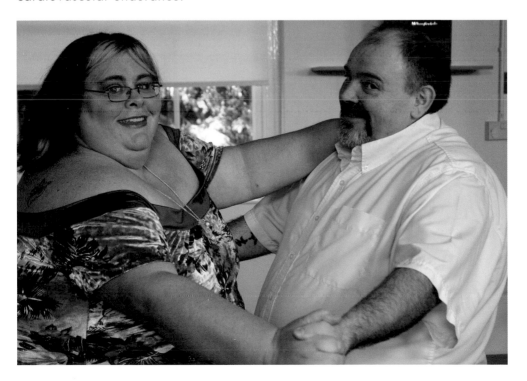

You can either do a dance exercise class or take more conventional dance lessons in ballroom, tap, jazz, street, salsa, Latin-American or even adult beginners' ballet! And belly-dancing is a wonderful exercise for women – all that hip-shaking and stomach-rolling really gets the muscles rippling.

Dance exercise will give a good workout, but all forms of dance will get you moving about. And you're never too old to hit the floor. Bruce Forsyth is till tap-dancing in his 80s! And it's been proven that the brain and body coordination required to dance can help ward off age-related conditions such as Alzheimer's.

Trampolining

You might buy one for the kids to use in the garden but there's not an adult in the country who wouldn't enjoy a bounce workout on a trampoline.

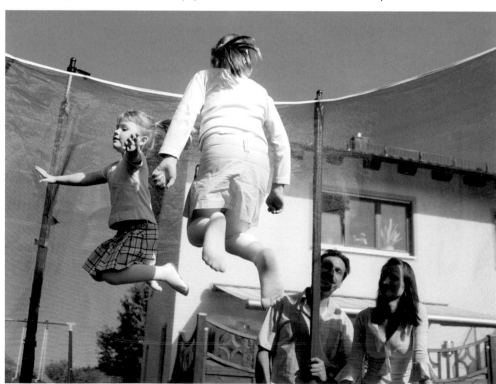

SAFETY

As with any equipment, you need to take extra care when children are using trampolines. With the large outdoor versions, make sure there is well-fitting and adequate padding around the edges, use a protective netting enclosure to stop bouncers flying off and don't let young children use it unsupervised. To avoid head clashes, only one person at a time should bounce on it.

Also, most trampolines have a weight restriction, so check the manufacturer's instructions.

It's good aerobic exercise, strenuous and repetitive, and although the impact on the joints is low because the web absorbs much of the shock, repeated low-level impact can be good for strengthening bones. It uses almost every muscle group in the body – legs, abdominals and arms – and improves coordination. Keeping your balance also strengthens those important core muscles. You can burn around 240 calories per hour trampolining (based on a person of 10 st 7 lb).

The different gravity effects (at the top of the bounce you are weightless, at the bottom you experience increased gravitational pull as you change direction) are also thought to stimulate the working of the lymph system. And it's such fun, you won't want to come off.

You can also buy mini-trampolines, called rebounders, which you can use inside the house. Some people swear by them to improve fitness and lymph draining (and even reduce cellulite!), while other people think they're a bit of a gimmick. But they can certainly be a useful addition to a home circuit, as you'll build up your heart rate in a 10-minute bouncing session. Vary the bounces using leg lifts, side leg lifts, twists and turns to get the most out of it.

Yoga/Pilates

There are many different sorts of yoga and Pilates classes, both private and at local gyms.

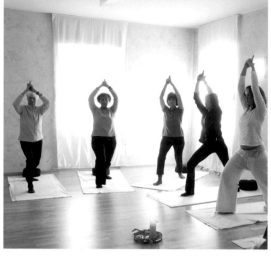

Yoga is especially good for improving flexibility and stretching, whereas Pilates specialises in strengthening the deep core muscles.

Most classes aren't designed to burn off lots of calories but they can be very useful for people who experience stiffness and back pain. They can improve posture and also have a very calming, de-stressing effect that some people find extremely helpful when making big life changes.

If you lack confidence in yourself, the breathing techniques and slow, gradual exercises can make you look at yourself in a more positive way.

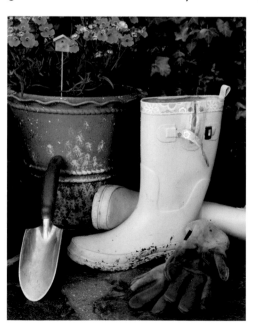

Housework/gardening

Okay, they're not Olympic events, but never forget that a bit of elbow grease burns calories too.

Digging the garden, weeding, mowing the lawn and planting pots all get the body bending and stretching, and have the added advantage of getting you outdoors in the fresh air.

Hoovering, ironing, changing the beds, dusting and washing up are also physical activities that will be doing their bit to burn calories. An hour of hoovering could burn around 193 calories per hour for a 12-stone woman, and dusting for an hour could burn 173 calories. And don't forget, mad though it may sound, you can always be exercising your body when you are standing still. When you're ironing or washing up, or even cleaning your teeth, you could be doing knee bends, or rising up on your toes to stretch leg muscles, or doing side leg lifts ...

Have you noticed how many advertising breaks there are in every commercial TV show? And hands up who sits staring at the screen for three minutes while they're on? It sounds extreme, but why not stand up and march on the spot through the ad breaks, or walk up and down the stairs a couple of times? You can build up lots of tiny little opportunities to keep moving instead of standing still. It all contributes to keeping those muscles working and, as we keep saying, a muscle burns more calories than fat.

Here are some more wasted moments when you could be walking on the spot – who cares what other people think if you're focused on your new life!

- Waiting for the bus or train
- Waiting for the kettle to boil
- Talking on a mobile phone
- Waiting for the kids outside school
- Watching the kids play in a sports match
- Waiting in a queue at the post office

Children and exercise

Young children are naturally bursting with energy that they need to run off. Watch little children in a park and often they just run around, pretending to be cars or horses, with nothing more sophisticated in mind than just running.

And they like nothing more than to have Mum or Dad or grandparents come to the park and push them on the swings or catch them at the bottom of the slide.

> **BURNING CALORIES**
>
> **What a 9.5 stone person burns in 30 minutes:**
>
> - **Running (6mph): 300 calories**
> - **Tennis (singles): 240 calories**
> - **Swimming (slow crawl): 240 calories**
> - **Cycling (12–14mph): 240 calories**
> - **Aerobic dancing: 195 calories**
> - **Brisk walking (4mph): 150 calories**
>
> Source: Department of Health, 2004

So although kids today say they like being in front of a computer screen, or watching TV, it's often because no one is offering them an alternative. We're all too nervous to give them the freedom to just disappear for the day on weekends, tearing back home when they're hungry.

So if they can't go out alone, then Mum and Dad are going to have to get out there with them and show them how to be active instead of couch potatoes. The most important thing is to make it fun.

A child may not want to swim 20 lengths of the local pool, but take them to a pool that has a slide, fountains and giant foam floats and they'll probably swim, dive and play happily for a couple of hours without feeling tired.

Roller-skating, ice-skating or bowling alleys are great places for a family day out, but if you don't want to spend money you can just organise a game of rounders in the local park. Tell them to bring some friends and then provide drinks and a couple of rugs to sit on.

Teenage girls in particular can be very resistant to exercise, worrying they don't look cool, but an hour's dance exercise in the right outfit is a great way to burn off flab.

Growing children are probably too young for strength training in a gym. Most local authority gyms won't let under-16s exercise there for insurance purposes, but you can certainly get them into mini-circuits at home.

Get bored teenagers to join a badminton class, or five-a-side football (boys and girls) or netball/basketball sessions.

But more important than anything, lead by example. Most overweight children have fat parents, don't forget, so if you sit in front of the TV all evening they are not going to see why they should get off their bottoms and move.

How much should I do?

It's easy to think you've done a week's worth of exercise with one intense visit to the gym or a long weekend walk. But exercise needs to be regular and spread throughout the week to have any effect on fitness and weight.

These are the minimum amounts of time needed to improve your fitness levels:

• Adults: 30 minutes of moderate-intensity physical activity at least five days a week.

• Children: 60 minutes of moderate-intensity physical activity every day.

Obese adults may need to do 60 to 90 minutes of exercise a day to combat their excess weight before they can do the maintenance programme of 30 minutes.

But it doesn't have to be done all in one go. Targets can be achieved with 10-minute bursts of activity spread throughout the day.

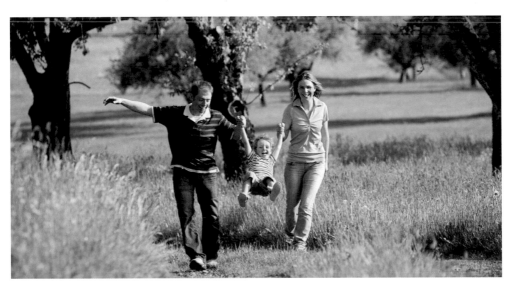

Other benefits of exercise

Improve your mood

Exercise has been proven to improve your mood and is now 'prescribed' by doctors as a treatment for mild depression. When you exercise, your body releases chemicals called endorphins, which act as mood-boosters, and they can give you a lift long after you stop moving.

When you next feel down, instead of reaching for the biscuit tin, go for a good brisk walk and you will almost certainly feel your spirits lift.

Strengthen your bones

Our bones are being remodelled all the time as bone is broken down and new bone is formed. Bones aren't solid, they're more like a honeycomb of cells that need to be renewed. They need calcium and vitamin D from a healthy diet but one of the most important things our bones need to keep them strong and keep replenishing themselves is exercise – and in particular what is called load-bearing or weight-bearing exercise. That means jogging, running, using the cross trainer or any exercise that puts some weighted pressure on the joints. It's thought that the action of the muscles against the joints promotes the formation of new bone.

It's especially important in women who have gone through the menopause, as lower oestrogen levels at this time can lead to thinning bones and eventually the serious disease of osteoporosis.

Do some weight-bearing exercise outdoors in the sunshine every day for a hit of bone-strengthening vitamin D and you'll double the benefits.

Improve your sleep

Many people claim they can't sleep well at night despite being tired, but doing regular exercise has been shown to improve the quality of sleep, which in turn

WORK IT OFF

A little snack surely can't hurt? Well, look at how hard you'll have to work to burn off these treats:

- A hot cross bun = 15 (men) to 20 (women) minutes' skipping
- One chocolate bar = 45 to 50 minutes' aquaerobics
- A fast-food burger with cheese = 70 to 85 minutes on the cross trainer
- One slice of fast-food pepperoni pizza = 40 to 45 minutes' swimming
- A 330 ml can of cola = 30 to 35 minutes on the rowing machine

As a rough calculation you need to burn 3,500 calories to lose one pound in weight. To lose one pound a week you need to cut down by 500 calories a day or, by upping your exercise level, you can cut back by 250 calories and burn an extra 250 calories, making a weekly total of 3,500.

So to lose two pounds a week you need to cut back or burn an extra 1,000 calories per day.

can help to regulate your weight. And no, not by stopping you popping to the fridge at midnight for a snack, but because our hormones are affected by our sleep patterns.

Earlier in the book (see page 12) we described how the hormone ghrelin stimulates your appetite and the hormone leptin tells you when you are full. But people with disturbed sleep often have higher levels of ghrelin and lower levels of leptin, so they feel hungrier even though they may have eaten plenty. In some American studies, men who were sleep deprived showed up to 45% increase in their desire for high-carbohydrate, energy-dense foods.

Very overweight people often suffer from sleep apnoea, a condition in which they stop breathing for a few seconds and then suddenly wake up, which seriously disturbs and reduces the quality of their sleep. Exercising and losing weight can improve these symptoms. Exercise has also been shown to improve the sleep patterns in people who suffer from restless legs at night.

Equipment

Although you can go to town and buy loads of fancy, expensive equipment, the good news is that, as detailed above, there's really no need to splash out. Just make sure you have the basics.

Heart-rate monitor

A heart-rate monitor measures your heart rate and alerts you to when your heart is working at the best rate for your sex, weight and age. There is a zone you're advised to stay within and most monitors will beep if you start working too hard or if you slacken off so that you're coasting. More sophisticated models will calculate the calories burned and can even estimate how many of those calories came from your body fat.

Most gyms will show you how to use a heart-rate monitor when you start before you spend money on one of your own.

Trainers

The days are long gone when you just went to buy a new pair of trainers – now the choice and price range are mind-blowing. But it's important to remember that technology and design have created trainers that are best for specific functions, so a tennis shoe will be very different in support and padding from a running shoe. A running shoe is designed for forward motion and has thicker heels and soles to help absorb shock and push the runner forward. An aerobics shoe has greater ankle support.

But unless you plan to take up one exercise seriously you should invest in the best quality all-round trainer or cross-trainer shoe and don't let the sales assistant bamboozle you with too much detail. The shoe should have good cushioning on the sole and good support around the heel and ankle.

Don't focus too much on your stomach. It takes 250,000 abdominal crunches to burn a pound of fat! Work the fat off first before you worry about a six-pack.

HOW MUCH? HOW OFTEN?

How many times a week should you do muscle-based exercise such as circuit training? As a guide, follow the muscular endurance FITT principle, which stands for:

- **F**requency: two to three times per week
- **I**ntensity: 40 to 50% of each muscle group
- **T**ime: variable depending on how many muscle groups are worked in each session (which, in this case, is 12 to 15 reps, one to two sets per exercise)
- **T**ype: variable but at least two exercises for each muscle group using slow and controlled form

Cardio fitness and weight control recommendations of aerobic exercise should be performed three to five days a week for 20 to 60 minutes at an intensity that achieves 55 to 90% of MHR (maximum heart rate).

WATER

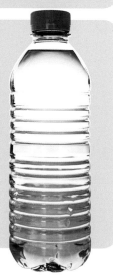

It's terribly important to drink enough water when you start exercising, both before and after your workout. Inadequately hydrated muscles weaken and cramp more quickly, so keep up your fluid levels during the day.

Unless you're exercising to a professional level, don't bother with special, over-hyped sports-energy drinks. Not only are they full of additives and sweeteners – the only pounds they'll help you lose are from your bank account!

Exercise

The Turner family from Barry

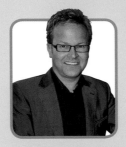

Steve visited the Turners from Barry, south Wales.

'I was meeting a bunch of beached blubber bellies who'd been gorging on grub for years. This bunch of pie munchers could eat their way through a mountain of food at mealtimes. They weren't in denial about how overweight they were but they yo-yo dieted and did absolutely no exercise at all. They'd actually got a treadmill but it was never used!'

The stats (after eight weeks)

Dad: **Dave**
Age: **43**
Height: **6' 2"**
Start weight: **23 st 10 lb**
Now weighs: **19 st**

Total weight loss: **4 st 10lb**

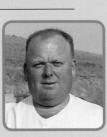

Mum: **Keri**
Age: **45**
Height: **5' 3"**
Start weight : **21 st 2 lb**
Now weighs: **18 st 2 lb**

Total weight loss: **3 st**

Daughter-in-law: **Sadie**
Age: **25**
Height: **5' 1"**
Start weight: **14 st 5 lb**
Now weighs: **11 st 6lb**

Total weight loss: **2 st 13 lb**

Total family weight loss: **10 st 9 lb**

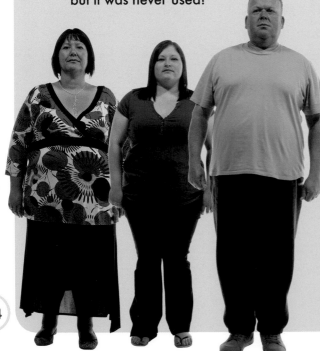

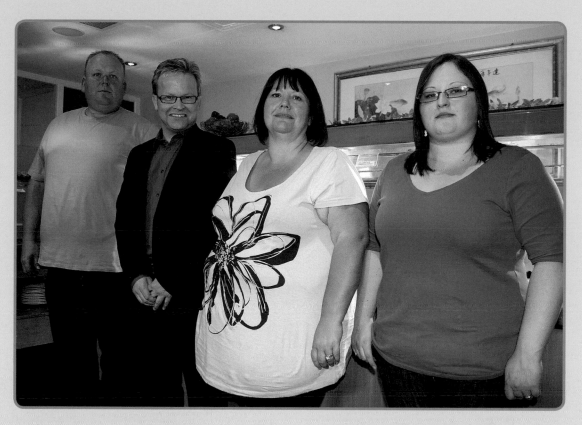

Main problem

Debt collector Keri was the classic yo-yo dieter who had tried every diet going, from Atkins to weight-loss pills, but although she was capable of shifting the weight it always went back on. She had a very sweet tooth, especially for chocolate, and did no exercise at all – she'd sometimes spend Sundays doing nothing. Her doctor had warned her that she was pre-diabetic but although she claimed she liked cooking, the family lived mainly off convenience foods. But she did cook big pies and loved feeding family and friends.

Scaffolding supervisor Dave wasn't a fan of doctors since he was diagnosed with very high blood pressure nearly 18 years ago and was prescribed medication for it. He did no exercise, ate convenience foods with Keri and liked his cans of lager and flagons of cold cider. He also drank masses of black coffee, which got his heart pumping.

Clerical officer Sadie admits she was lazy and preferred convenience foods to proper meals. She was a snacker throughout the day, although she'd tried diets before. 'I couldn't do it on my own – I got bored.'

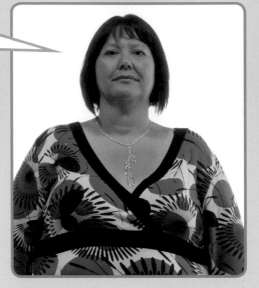

Keri: 'I was a big fat faker.'

Main motivation

Health was a serious concern for all the Turners and Steve's shock tactic of taking them to a coffin warehouse really brought home to the family how they were gambling with their lives. Dave had been the subject of cruel comments about his weight but it took a real eye-opener like this to bring home to him what risks he was taking.

Keri had been warned before about her health and she thought that the pressure of appearing on TV would be a great motivation to lose the weight.

Sadie was extremely disturbed by the coffins and freaked out. Her dad had a stroke at a young age and her mum had been diagnosed with diabetes – both weight-related problems. As well as her health risks, Sadie was worried that her ever-increasing weight would make it difficult or risky for her to have children – and make her a poor role model as a mum.

Typical day's food: Keri

Breakfast:	Almond croissant, cappuccinos with sugar
Mid-morning:	Crisps, Coke, chocolate
Lunch:	Sandwich, crisps, Coke, cappuccinos
Dinner:	Full Indian or Chinese takeaway, or pizza

Keri drank up to six takeaway cappuccinos a day with two sugars each and Dave drank up to 15 black coffees a day with sugar. One teaspoon of sugar is 15 calories, so Dave was taking in an extra 225 calories just in sugar, along with a huge amount of caffeine.

Medical tests

Consultant surgeon Chris Pring ran tests on the Turners that showed:

Keri: knew her tests would show up that she was pre-diabetic because her own doctor had warned her. She also had high cholesterol and blood pressure and her body was 54.8% fat. She was carrying 11 st 6 lb of fat!

Dave: Chris Pring was worried about Dave because his blood pressure was so dangerously high at 185/120 – high enough to be hospitalised. He was told that he had to take exercising very gently at first because of the strain on his heart. His body was 56% fat – he was carrying 14 st 13 lb of fat.

Sadie: with her family history she was told she was 12 times more likely to get diabetes than someone without her risks. She was carrying a lot of abdominal fat and her cholesterol was higher than the healthy range. Her body was 44.1% fat so she was carrying an extra 6 st 4 lb of fat.

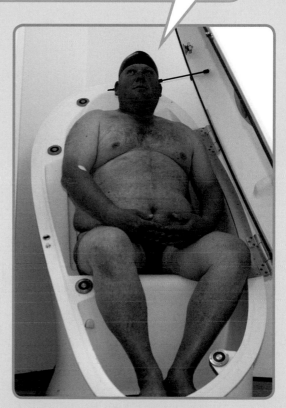

Dave: 'The lads on site called me Rhino, I was so big. I'd like them to call me whippet instead!'

Lifestyle changes

Dave's high blood pressure wasn't something he could ignore any longer or control just through medication. All the Turners were facing health crises. They had to lose weight, and quickly, but more importantly they had to find a way to keep it off. No more yo-yo dieting, this needed a total change of lifestyle with no room for slipping back. They had to stop eating all the pies, start walking – and they had to admit how unhappy being overweight was making them.

Steve said, 'They all told me that they put on fake smiles on the outside but are unhappy inside. But I can't wave a magic wand.'

They needed to:

1. Start cooking and think about what they were eating instead of eating and drinking from habit
2. Plan meals in advance
3. Take time over eating so they were having proper meals instead of just eating all day
4. Build exercise into their daily lives

Exercise regime

Dave's high blood pressure meant he had to monitor carefully what he did to begin with. Walking would be the key to kick-starting his weight loss.

Personal trainer Chris Jones started them on the treadmill at home and gave them targets to walk outdoors – luckily they live in a beautiful place!

'Dave needed to start gently but I was impressed by how committed and motivated they all were. I used the bike in the gym because it takes some of the weight and protects the joints from stress, and I introduced some interval training so they would work harder for very short bursts. This helps to burn the fat. As the weight dropped off and, even better, Dave's blood pressure started to come down, I could introduce some circuits; just two to begin with then upped it to four or five.

'They have done amazingly well and I think Sadie was my real surprise. Her fitness levels have gone through the roof; she really pushed herself and her whole shape has changed. They've had their ups and downs like everyone but I'm really impressed at what they've achieved.'

Keri admits that she will never enjoy going to the gym. She does the circuits with Chris, using the cross trainer and bike, but what she has discovered instead is a love of walking. She, Dave and Sadie will walk for an hour along the cliffs of Barry without thinking of it as exercise and every Sunday she and Sadie

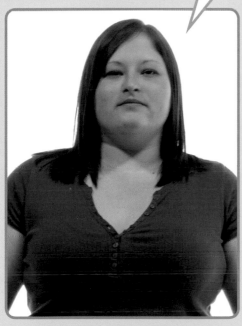

Sadie: 'I was everybody's fat friend but I felt like a fat ugly pretender who was just putting it on for show.'

go swimming and they do a weekly aquaerobics class. They also run around a local park.

Dave has transformed his whole routine. He began by walking on a treadmill in the house and hasn't stopped since the first day. He gets up an hour earlier every day to walk on the treadmill before work. He no longer drives the company van to work but walks 20 minutes down to his workmate's house to get a lift. After work he asks to be dropped off on the outskirts of Barry and he walks the 45-minute journey home. Then on the weekends and some evenings he'll go walking by the sea with Keri and Sadie.

Sadie admits that she used to be so lazy she wouldn't even walk the few minutes from her house to work. But once she started she wasn't going to be a quitter.

'I don't believe in giving 90%. Yes, I've had a few low points but because we do it together there's always someone to drag you out. My whole attitude has changed; I'm more confident and I don't care what anyone says about me. I've lived here for about seven years and I didn't know half the places – it's a beautiful place to walk around.'

Healthy eating

Nutritionist Jessica Wilson said, 'The Turners are a fabulous family who took everything on board. They were terrible snackers but understood that they needed to eat proper meals and in small portions. They knew what they should be doing – and they've replaced all the unhealthy stuff with fresh vegetables

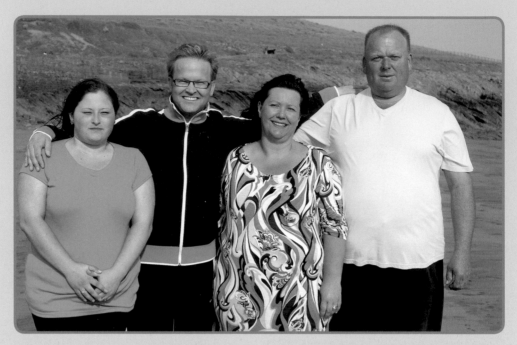

and fruit. And they plan ahead – one of the best ways to stop falling into bad habits.'

Keri has found that planning her meals has made the biggest difference and she takes all her own food into work instead of grazing from the vending machine.

'I have half a grapefruit before work and then when I get in I'll have a low-fat cereal with skimmed milk. At about 11am I have an apple and for lunch I have a home-made salad. I don't take any bread in and I don't have any more fizzy cola drinks. In the evening I usually have some fish with salad or vegetables.

'One of the biggest things I gave up were my daily cappuccinos – I could have up to six a day. After Steve pointed out that I could be eating five doughnuts every time I had a coffee, I swapped to fruit teas. I did get a bit of coffee withdrawal but I drank lots of water instead.

'We can't believe the money we are saving by eating healthily! Dave would sometimes have five black coffees and a fried egg sandwich before work but now has a healthy breakfast.

'Sadie plans out seven days' meals before she does the weekly food shop and she takes her own lunch to work.

'I cook fresh food every day and I know there's no last-minute grabbing of stuff in the fridge.'

Progress highs and lows

Dave nearly dropped out of the show before it started. 'I thought it would be all about doctors and I didn't want to make all these changes, I knew I had high blood pressure. But Phil Huzzey (see page 64), who was in the first series of the show, called me. He had had a heart attack, and losing weight and taking exercise completely changed his life so he inspired me to carry on.

'I remember on the weekend of the second week I was doing some work over at my parents' house and really wanted some icy-cold cider they had, but I looked at the label and thought what calories I would be taking in and thought, "No, I won't."

'I can do that now – look at pork pies and things in the supermarket and think it's just not worth it.

'I think having the camera forcing me to face up to what I'd done to myself was a low moment too.'

Keri: 'The hard part has been stopping using sweets and chocolate as an emotional crutch, especially when I had PMS. If I feel bloated and miserable I'm used to grabbing something chocolatey to give me a lift but when you look at a chocolate bar and think – that would take me three hours in the gym to work off – it doesn't seem so tempting!'

Sadie: 'Steve bought me a dress I really liked but he bought it two sizes too small to encourage me through the tough days. It's actually too big now, which gives me a real buzz!'

The family says:

Dave: 'When I started this my blood pressure was dangerously high; when I went to my GP the other day my blood pressure was 132/77. That's back down to normal. My GP literally almost fell off his chair! I can't tell you what that means. I went on this programme because I wanted to stay alive. I know Keri has tried to lose weight in the past and I thought I supported her but I'd come in on a Friday night, have a few cans

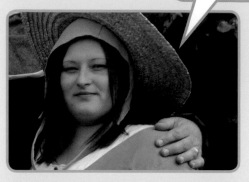

Sadie: 'I would love to walk down the beach and feel sexy for once.'

of lager and have no idea of what the calorie or fat content of the food I was eating was. But now we really support each other. I can be a big baby sometimes and throw my toys out of the pram but Keri and Sadie are there to keep me going and if they've had a good week I'll send them a text saying "Well done" or buy them some flowers.

'We get so much more out of life now. We still have a good social life but we don't have to go over the top. Our families and friends are right behind us and they ask us over to parties just the same.

'Losing weight is fantastic but having my health back after 18 years of medication is what really matters.'

Keri: 'I've been back to my doctor and in the space of eight weeks my blood sugar is normal and my cholesterol is down from 5.7 to 4.9. I'm off my medication and I feel so much fitter.

'I would never have thought just eight weeks ago that I could find time to go swimming and do aquaerobics but now I love it. Sadie and I have always been close but this has made us even closer.

'Having the support of Dave and Sadie has made this so much easier – to be honest, I haven't found it hard at all. I've had just one friend I had to drop because she wasn't encouraging me but there's another one that I can email when I'm tempted and ask him to talk me out of it!

'Every milestone you pass feels amazing. I did the 5K Cancer Research Race for Life last year. Before that I couldn't walk down the street without needing a rest. We do so much more and I feel so much healthier.

'Jessica opened my eyes to cooking and I bought a new cookbook.

'Now I can start buying clothes in normal shops – I bought a dress from George at ASDA and even found a dress in Tesco that was too big!

'My self-confidence is so much higher – I put on a happy face before

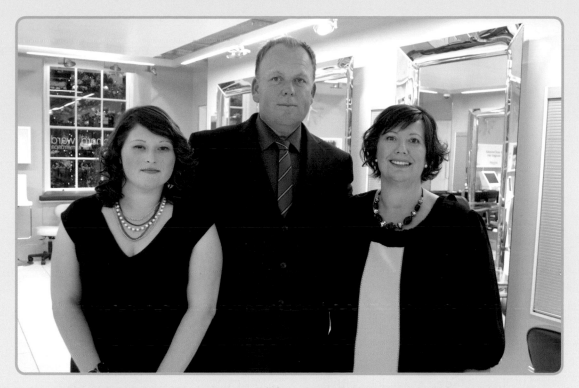

when really I was so unhappy with my weight.'

Sadie: 'I've booked a summer holiday and I feel confident that I'll be wearing a bikini after years of covering up with a sarong! This has brought us all even closer than we were and I feel so much better about myself.'

The Turner family's top tips

- People can be cruel if you're fat but keep your chin up and remember you can do it.

- Keep a food diary and be honest about what you eat.

- Watch the drinks – those coffees really add up!

- Start walking – just get off your bottom and walk!

- Set progressive goals and when you achieve them, set another. Don't set a huge one that will dishearten you if you don't reach it.

ANOTHER COFFEE?

Just look at how the fat in coffee adds up:

- 1 large cappuccino = 9.3 g of fat = 7 tins of rice pudding

- 1 large latte = 15 g of fat = 1 portion of chips

- 1 large mocha = 26.6 g of fat

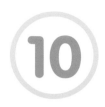

Q&As

You should now have all the information and motivation you need to start your family's new lifestyle. If you feel yourself slipping back into your old ways, then reread the sections on motivation or look at the stories of the families from the show. They prove that, with some hard work, dedication and the support of your family, you really can get fantastic results. Don't forget to keep encouraging each other in your journey to health and fitness – a bit of competition can really help you on your way.

There will always be a few difficulties in your dieting journey, so here are some essential troubleshooting Q&As that address some of the queries you might have once you've started your new way of life.

Healthy eating

Q **I'm trying to wean my kids off their favourite fast-food pizzas and burgers, but they refuse to eat any vegetables. How can I get them to eat them?**

A Sounds sneaky, but at the beginning it's a good idea to hide them in other foods. A pasta sauce, for example, doesn't have to be just tomato, you can liquidise carrots into it and some pumpkin, red peppers or squash. Chilli con carne or shepherd's pie is a great place to hide some pea purée or you can add almost anything to a soup, then blend out the lumps.

Get them used to new tastes – carrot is naturally sweet – before you try vegetables in their own right. But one of the best ways to get kids to eat is to let them help you in the kitchen. According to the British Food Council, children are more willing to eat food they have chosen themselves, so take them to the shops and let them experiment in the kitchen with you.

If they're very young, just coming up with new sandwich ideas can be fun, or get them used to using carrot and cucumber sticks with dips. Encourage them to use a 'rainbow chart' and see if they can eat a vegetable of every colour every day. And don't forget, a home-made pizza can be loaded with fresh vegetables and not full of fat. Let them choose from fresh toppings and make their own.

But most of all, stay calm, eat loads of veggies yourself, eat with them and eventually they will follow you.

Q **My son wants the same lunch box for school meals every day and I'm worried he doesn't get enough variety. He has a plain cheese sandwich on white bread, a packet of crisps, a carton of blackcurrant juice and a chocolate biscuit. The school wants us to change to healthy eating but I'm worried it will come back uneaten.**

A There's nothing more disheartening than opening a lunch box when your child gets home and finding food not eaten. Simple little steps rather than a dramatic overhaul is best.

Swap the white bread for wholemeal – maybe use one of the half-and-half breads to start. Or try using wholemeal pitta pockets, as something new may be more acceptable. Swap the carton of blackcurrant for very diluted blackcurrant squash or other juice – pop it in the freezer for a while before school and it will still be cold. Instead of a biscuit, give him a small carton of fruit – berries in season or grapes or satsuma segments can be eaten with fingers. Drop the crisps and try him with breadsticks, or make crisps a Friday treat.

And ask him to choose a different salad to go with his cheese sandwich every day. If he doesn't want a tomato in the sandwich (it can make the sandwich soggy), pop a couple of sweet cherry tomatoes in separately.

It won't work overnight, but children are surprisingly adaptable when there's nothing else on offer. And if it isn't eaten and he comes home hungry, don't 'reward him' for not eating by offering him unhealthy snacks – offer hummus and pitta bread, fruit or wholemeal toast.

Q My husband loves spicy tastes and smothers most of his food in black pepper! I'm trying to cut back on salt when I cook, so should I make him cut back on pepper?

A No! Unlike salt, which isn't good in large amounts, pepper has health benefits, not least that it helps you to absorb the nutrients in your food. Turmeric, an Indian spice with wonderful anti-inflammatory properties, isn't absorbed at all well unless it's eaten with black pepper. This is because black pepper contains something called piperine, which helps the absorption process. So ditch the salt and embrace the pepper!

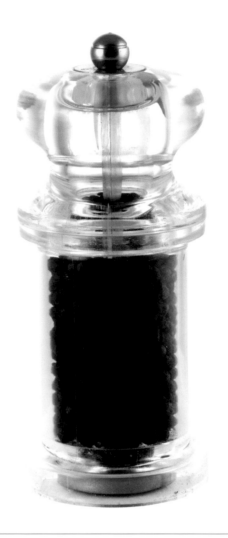

Q I'm trying to eat whole-grain rice instead of white rice but a friend says that white basmati rice is good for you. I hate whole-grain rice with curries, so can I go back to white rice?

A As a rule of thumb, always choose whole-grain over refined rice and yes, basmati is a refined rice. But it actually has a slightly lower starch content and a lower GI than other white rice so is a better choice.

You can get brown basmati, which would be the best compromise, but white basmati is better than regular white rice if you must have it with your curries!

Q I'm trying to drink 1.2 litres of water a day but find it a struggle and am always going to the loo at work. Is it really necessary?

A Most of us don't drink enough water so recommending six to eight glasses is a big step for most people. However, you may be getting an adequate fluid intake from other sources – teas, fruit juice, coffees, etc., so what you should be doing is swapping some of these for water instead of adding water to your current supply. Add lemon or lime slices to take away the blandness or try naturally carbonated mineral waters for a change. You can tell if you aren't drinking enough as your urine will be darker than a pale-straw colour.

Q I'm trying to eat more substantial breakfasts but I'm worried that eggs are high in cholesterol and I should avoid them.

A There was a scare about the cholesterol content of eggs some years ago and the advice was to eat just a couple a week. Thankfully research was done into how eggs affect the cholesterol levels in the blood and the advice now is that it is quite safe to eat eggs without worrying about any change in your cholesterol levels.

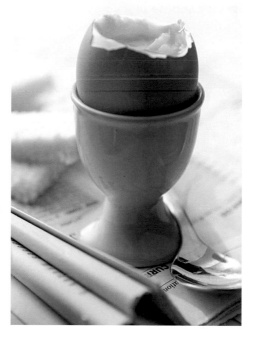

The important thing is how you eat them – poached or boiled eggs are healthy (and scrambled if you don't load them with butter). They are a great start to the day, especially if you have a glass of fresh orange juice with them, which helps the body to absorb the iron in them. But avoid fried eggs – all that grease!

Q I keep reading about grains like quinoa and I've seen them in the supermarket but I don't know what to do with them and whether they are really any better for me.

A Quinoa (pronounced *keen-wah*) is a really healthy food as it has a very high level of protein and is a source of manganese, iron, B vitamins and vitamin E, which makes it a good choice for vegetarians. As it is technically a seed rather than a grain, it is a good source of fatty acids, such as linoleic and oleic acids.

You simply rinse it well, bring it to the boil and simmer for about 15 minutes. It fluffs up and has a slightly nutty texture and flavour but absorbs the flavours of sauces and casseroles beautifully.

You can even have it with some fruit and nuts for breakfast. Store it in an airtight container, preferably in the fridge. Buy some today!

Q Why do you keep recommending nuts when they are full of fat?

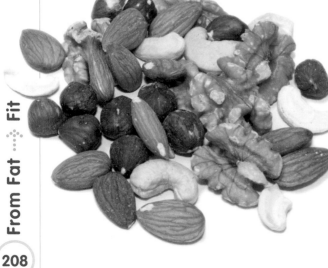

A It's true nuts have a high fat content but they are a good source of the essential fatty acids we need for our health. They also have lots of other health benefits that outweigh their high calorie/fat content. No one is suggesting you should eat bagfuls of them, but a handful added to a bowl of fruit or porridge gives a good protein portion. Almonds, walnuts and brazil nuts are good choices. What you should avoid are the roasted, coated nuts as snacks.

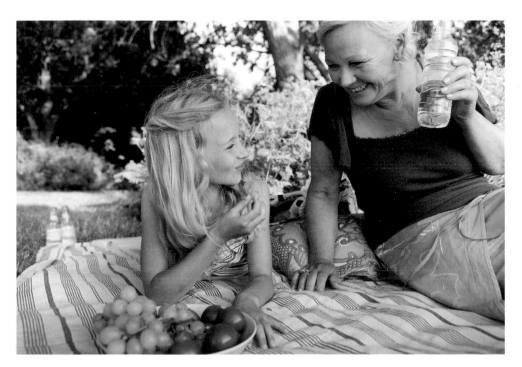

Q I'm confused. Some people say you should eat three good meals a day with no snacking in between, other people tell me to eat little and often to keep my blood-sugar level constant. I'm not too sure what to do.

A Most nutritionists agree that you shouldn't go more than three to four hours without eating something (unless you're asleep!). But that doesn't mean eating a bag of crisps or a packet of biscuits between meals – a piece of fruit is ideal.

The structure of your day should be three meals and you shouldn't skip one – especially breakfast.

Try to include protein with carbohydrates at meal times as it slows down the speed at which you absorb carbs. Bulk up your meals with lots of vegetables – they fill you up and are packed with vitamins.

Exercise

Q I'm exercising quite hard every day but as soon as I get home I'm starving and seem to be eating twice as much as before! I'm worried I'll end up putting on weight as my loss on the scales has slowed down.

A It's understandable that your body needs extra fuel if you're exercising hard but there are several questions here. Are you sure you're drinking enough water? Sometimes we confuse hunger with thirst, especially after exercising. Are you eating the right things after exercising? Exercise uses up glycogen stores, and studies show that a combination of carbohydrate and protein eaten within two hours of exercise is the best way to restore glycogen reserves and to help repair any muscle wear and tear. Try eating a chicken, turkey or salmon wholemeal sandwich maybe, or scrambled eggs on toast – and see if that helps. Be careful that you're not simply listening to your brain tell you that you 'deserve' more food as a reward for exercise!

Q My husband and I have started going to the gym, where a trainer has recommended we use some weights for resistance work. But my husband is worried that I'll develop pronounced muscles on my arms and thighs if I do weights and says I should stick to running.

A Women often think that if they use weights they'll end up looking like a bodybuilder, but it's not true. Women's muscle tone is different to men's because they have less of the hormone testosterone, which gives men their bulkier shape. Use light weights with lots of repetitions and you'll find that your muscles develop that lean, toned look without adding bulk. It's particularly important to do this as you lose weight so you build tone where fat used to be.

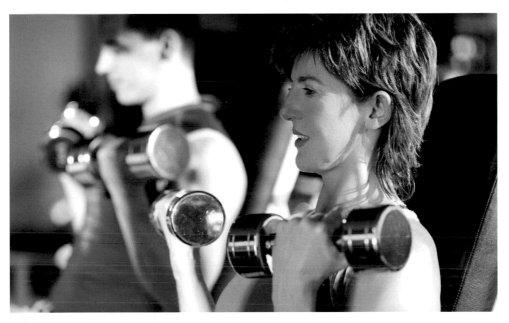

Q I lost a lot of weight in order to get pregnant and now I am having a baby, I'm terrified I'll pile it all back on. I'm scared to keep exercising but if I sit at home while my husband goes running or to the gym, which we used to do together, I think I'll start eating biscuits again!

A The first thing is to check with your doctor whether there are any medical reasons why you shouldn't be exercising – a history of miscarriage or anaemia, for example, might suggest that you should take it easy. But there are positive health benefits for you and the baby in keeping fit during pregnancy – and certainly for not piling the weight back on. Walking is great at any stage of pregnancy as long as you feel comfortable, and swimming is ideal as it takes the weight off your baby bump. Your local pool may well do special classes. Why not swim while your husband goes to the gym, or walk around the park while he does his running circuits?

The fitter you stay during pregnancy, the easier you'll find it to get fit after the baby is born.

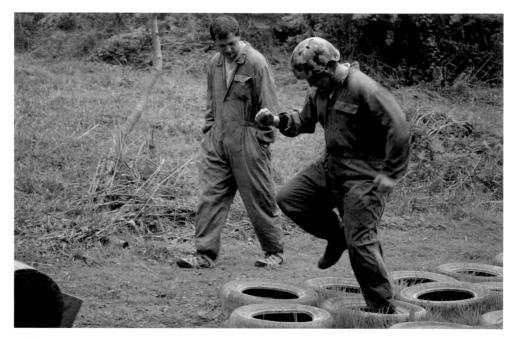

Q There's a gym at my new office and because my weekends are busy with the kids I've started doing intensive 60-minute workouts every lunch time. My wife says I'm overdoing it but I feel fine. Should I take a day off?

A Although exercising daily is great, if you're doing intense muscle work day after day, your muscles never get the chance to repair themselves, which can take up to 48 hours.

It sounds as though you're doing the same routine every day, so why not vary it so you aren't exercising the same muscle groups? And although you say you're busy with the kids on weekends, don't forget you can get a lot of exercise done by playing football in the park or taking them swimming or cycling.

It's important to show children that exercise is fun – not just all sweat in a gym – if you want them to be active too.

Q I've started exercising for the first time in my life – I'm 28. I've started going to the gym, using the rowing machine and bike, and doing circuits, and I swim once a week. Although the weight is starting to shift, my muscles are terribly sore and I'm scared that I've done some lasting damage. I do warm up well and cool down. Should I just try to work through it?

A Well, first off, well done for taking up exercise – it sounds a well-balanced programme.

However, it's possible that you may be suffering from Delayed Onset Muscle Soreness (DOMS). Taking up an intense exercise programme, or changing activities, can cause tiny tears in the muscle tissue or the tissue that surrounds it, and by continuing to exercise you never let the muscles repair themselves.

DOMS usually come on about 12 to 48 hours after exercise – unlike the immediate pain of a sprain or strain and the duller next-day ache of temporary muscle soreness you get when you push yourself a bit harder. The only real treatment is to rest for a while, then, when you restart exercising, take it more slowly and only gradually build up back to your current level.

It is quite common so don't be disheartened, but once you're feeling better remember that prevention is always better than cure. Some sufferers claim massage, ice baths or stretching helps but there's no one rule for all, I'm afraid.

If you've got to this section of the book, you should have a good overview of what you need to do to get slimmer and fitter – and how to motivate yourself and your family to achieve those goals.

If you feel yourself slipping back into your old ways, then reread the sections on motivation or look at the inspirational stories of the families from the show. They prove that, with some hard work, dedication and the support of your family, you really can get fantastic results. Don't forget to keep encouraging each other in your journey to health and fitness – a bit of competition can really help you on your way.

Resources

We'd like to thank all the experts who have offered their advice to our families. If you'd like to find out more about any aspect of improving your families health and fitness levels, these website addresses might be useful.

Our experts

Steve Miller
Steve is a specialist business and lifestyle motivator. For more advice on his motivational work, please visit:
www.themotivationhouse.com

Nutritionists

Professor David McCarthy
David is Professor of Human Nutrition at London Metropolitan University.
www.londonmet.ac.uk

Jessica Wilson, Dip ION, mBANT, NTCC
Jessica is a fully qualified nutritionist and television producer and has worked as a consultant on both series of *Fat Families*.
www.taitnutrition.com, **info@taitnutrition.com**

Personal trainers

Russell Byham
Russell is a fully qualified personal fitness trainer based in Essex. He offers one-to-one and group training.
www.russellbyham.com

Dave Coard

Dave is an ABA Coach, British Boxing Board of Control Coach, Boxercise Coach, SAQ/YMCA Personal Trainer, ISRM gym instructor and BFT Coach (Triathlon), and is based in Luton.

www.boxfit.org.uk

Chris O'Hanlon

Chris is a fully qualified personal trainer and sports therapist based in Bedfordshire.

www.chrisohanlon.co.uk

Dawn Jolleys

Dawn is a fully qualified personal trainer and obesity consultant based in Wiltshire.

dawn.jolleys@nuffieldhealth.com

Chris Jones

Chris Jones is a fully qualified personal trainer based in Glamorgan, south Wales.

www.jonestraining.co.uk

Bernie Saupe

Bernie is a fully qualified personal trainer based in Portsmouth, offering all-round fitness training, boxercise and nutritional advice.

www.gtxfitness.co.uk

Health charities and websites

British Heart Foundation

This charity provides information about the risks, causes and management of heart disease.

www.bhf.org.uk

Main tel: 020 7554 0000, heart helpline: 0300 330 3311, internet@bhf.org.uk

British Nutrition Foundation

A charity providing excellent information on all aspects of food and nutrition, from children to adults.

www.nutrition.org.uk

Tel: 020 7404 6504, postbox@nutrition.org.uk

High Holborn House, 52–54 High Holborn, London WC1V 6RQ

Change4Life

This public health programme from the Department of Health has lots of ideas for getting the family up and moving and eating healthily.

www.nhs.uk/change4life

Tel: 0300 123 4567

Diabetes UK

This charity specialises in the prevention and management of diabetes.

www.diabetes.org.uk

Tel: 020 7424 1000, info@diabetes.org.uk

Macleod House, 10 Parkway, London NW1 7AA

H.E.A.R.T UK

This charity raises awareness about the risks of high cholesterol and provides information on lowering cholesterol levels.

www.heartuk.org.uk

Helpline tel: 0845 450 5988, ask@heartuk.org.uk

7 North Road, Maidenhead, Berkshire, SL6 1PE

Patient UK

A useful health website with information provided by doctors and nurses on a range of health issues, including healthy eating and exercise.

www.patient.co.uk

The Vegan Society

This educational charity provides useful recommendations on how to achieve a balanced diet with no animal-sourced products.

www.vegansociety.com

Tel: 0121 523 1730, info@vegansociety.com

Donald Watson House, 21 Hylton Street, Hockley, Birmingham B18 6HJ

The Vegetarian Society

This educational charity encourages a vegetarian lifestyle and has good advice on eating a balanced meat-free diet.

www.vegsoc.org

Tel: 0161 925 2000, info@vegsoc.org

Parkdale, Dunham Road, Altrincham, Cheshire, England WA14 4QG

Weight Loss Resources

This weight-loss programme provides calorie and nutritional information, and you can check the calorific content of most everyday foods here.

www.weightlossresources.co.uk

Tel: 01733 345592, helpteam@weightlossresources.co.uk

29 Metro Centre, Woodston, Peterborough, PE2 7UH

Find out more about exercise

Swimming

Your local authority swimming pool should have a timetable of swimming lessons and sessions, but for more information on any aspect of swimming visit:

www.swimming.org

www.welshasa (Wales)

www.scottishswimming.com (Scotland)

Cycling

Your local authority leisure service should have information on cycle paths and trails near you but for more information on cycling visit:

www.britishcycling.org.uk / www.keepfit.org.uk

SKY TV also run group rides for all abilities throughout the country, led by professional cyclists. They are run at local levels but also in major cities. For details of rides in your areas visit:

www.goskyride.com

Rope skipping

Rope skipping is great exercise on your own, and even better in a group! For news about skipping events and team coaching visit:

www.brsa.org.uk

Dance classes

You can join classes with a partner or do ballet, tap street, jazz or line dancing on your own. There are many dance associations and classes around the UK, but you can try these websites as a starting point:

www.britishcouncil.org/arts-dance

www.dancesport.uk.com (specialises in ballroom, Latin Amercian, salsa, tango and other forms of partnered dance)

Gym work

Private gyms and health clubs generally have an excellent range of equipment and trainers but so do most local authority-run gyms, which are a cheaper alternative. Find information on gyms and leisure centres in your local area, see you local authority website. Look for off-peak memberships, family deals or concessions, which are cheaper still.

Index

Acknowledgements

This book couldn't have been written without the brave and determined people who tried and tested the advice – the families. Thank you all for your honesty, hard work and sense of humour – you have truly inspired others and proved that families really do stick together through thick and thin!

Thanks to all the personal trainers who put them through their paces and offered their time and expertise in helping write the exercise chapters. We're hugely grateful to obesity expert Professor David McCarthy and London Metropolitan University, the source of the medical wisdom and advice. And the tastiest section of the book is down to nutritionist Jessica Wilson, who contributed the delicious recipes and dietary advice.

Thank you to the show's stylists and to leading hair guru Richard Ward and all his team, and the team from Lockonego. Behind the scenes of the show, there is a truly hard working and dedicated team led by series producer Paul Tasker and unit manager Janine Terry. Also behind the scenes are Steve Miller's amazing assistant Terry, agents Sian Smyth and Eddie Bell, as well as our book agent Clare Hulton. Thank you all.

Huge thanks to Stuart Murphy, Celia Taylor, Siobhan Mulholland, Emma Read and the team from Sky1 for their support, encouragement and positivity.

Thanks to the inspirational energy centre who is Steve Miller. Everyone who has come into contact with Steve has benefitted from his passion and drive to help others succeed in their goals. Thank you Steve.

And a special thanks to Sally Morris for combining everything from the show to write this book.

– Laura Mansfield, Executive Producer, Outline Productions